MW00711026

the
heart of
living well

six principles

for a life of

health,

beauty,

and balance

judy lubin, MPH

heart and style books

© 2007 by Judy M. Lubin

A Heart and Style Books First Edition

All rights reserved. No part of this book may be reproduced, stored in a retrieval system, or transmitted in any form, by any means, including mechanical, electric, photocopying, recording or otherwise, without the prior written permission of the publisher

Library of Congress Preassigned Control Number: 2007933538
ISBN: 978-0-615-15139-7
Cover design: Brand Navigation and Jenny Mac Design
Interior design: Jenny Mac Design
Author photo: Jessica Garris-Scott

The material in this book is provided for information only and should not be construed as medical or psychological advice or instruction. It is sold with the understanding that the author and publisher shall have neither liability nor responsibility for any injury caused or alleged to be caused directly or indirectly by the information presented in this book. Always consult with your physician or other appropriate health professionals for recommendations appropriate to your specific needs.

Heart and Style Books
Heart and Style Media
A division of JML Communications Group, LLC
Rockville, MD

Printed in the United States of America

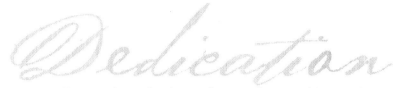

Dedication

To grandma, thank you for your love and inspiration.

To my mother and the family of women who touched and shaped my life, I am forever grateful for your love, guidance and support.

And to all women who yearn for health, beauty, balance and wholeness, may this work inspire and inform your journey.

contents

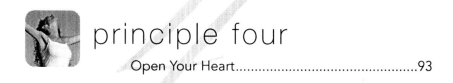

principle four

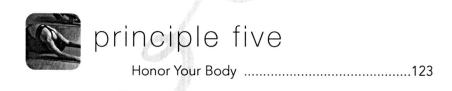

principle five

principle six

Introduction

Wellness—a higher calling

Everyone, from New Age gurus to fitness experts to gourmet chefs, tells us of the joys of living well. When you hear it coming from so many disparate corners, it can start to feel like living well is just some nebulous concept. Yet, we all want to live well. But what does it really mean? For most women, living well is living at our most optimal state of being, in balance and in harmony with ourselves and others. After years of personal exploration and work guiding others, I have come to believe that wellness is a lifelong, holistic path toward achieving that balance and harmony. It is a unique expression of mind, body, heart and spirit—more than just being healthy, true wellness is about being whole and complete.

Because of stress, painful life experiences, disability or illness, you may believe that you will never experience wellness. But wellness is not something way out in the ether, untouchable and unattainable. It is inside of you, right now, waiting for you to open to it.

wellness is a practice

Wellness, at its core, is about living a conscious life in line with our values. It is not only an ideal but a practice. We practice wellness by learning to make choices that are aligned with the truth of who we are—divine beings with a divine destiny. At times we may falter or stray off the path, but our love for our self calls us back. While life is fluid, ever-evolving and challenging, our longing for wellness is constant. The call comes from a place deep inside, from our spirit, the center of our being. Spirit calls us to be healthier, to seek fulfillment and to express our highest self.

Your spirit is always connected to the goodness within yourself and to the creative power of the universe—you might call this power God, Divine, Spirit, Source or by some other name (I use these interchangeably throughout the book). Whatever concept or being you recognize, at the most basic level, wellness is a spiritual path.

Spirit invites and beckons us to live a life of health, beauty and harmony through choices and practices that enrich, enlighten and empower our lives. When we eat for vitality, move our bodies for energy, pray for health and sleep for rest, we engage in sacred practices that honor the love and wisdom with which we were created.

Good health is physical and psychological vitality, a passion and enthusiasm that lead to an overall sense of wellness and gratitude for the blessings in life.

—ANDREA SULLIVAN, N.D.

We women are wonderfully complex and beautiful. Inside each of us are natural rhythms, energies and instincts that direct us to our best and healthiest life—if we are willing to listen. However, the rapid pace of everyday life, societal pressure, media messages and emotional traumas have caused the majority of women to tune out many of these natural abilities. But we can learn to trust ourselves again by making choices that are aligned with our deepest desires to be whole, happy and well.

Although I have worked in the health field for nearly ten years as a researcher, educator, writer, weight loss consultant, coach and advocate, I have not always thought of health as a transformative tool. I always believed health was the foundation for a good life but never thought of the pursuit of health and wellness as a transformative path in the way that I have just described. As I have traveled my own journey toward healing and wellness and supported other women on their own voyages of discovery, my perspective has changed.

I watch many women struggle to make lifestyle changes, only to hit emotional and mental roadblocks. Stress is the biggest culprit, but the inability to face underlying fears equally hinders success. Most recently, as designer and director of a lifestyle coaching program, I watched women walk away from the opportunity to change their lives, even though the coaching service was offered *free of charge*. There were all types of excuses: *I don't have time right now. This is not what I expected. I'm not ready for this.* We all have the right to change our mind about a decision that we discover is not right for us, but there was something else going on. Some of the women were "not ready" for coaching. The program asked them to be accountable for their lives, and some of us just aren't ready to do that. But it is that discomfort that usually moves us to action. When we decide that we are so tired, so fed up, so unhappy with the way we are feeling or living, we make a commitment to overhaul our lives and stop making excuses.

I was also surprised that many women, even some of those who completed the program, expressed a desire to have someone "tell me what to do." Aside from much-needed support and specific recommendations, such as what to eat for heart health or cancer prevention, I believe that most of us already know how to be well—we have an internal guide to steer us in the right direction. That guide is our spirit. Our failure to make this vital connection to our source of inner wisdom and energy is the missing link in our attempts to live well.

In the forthcoming pages you'll find a variety of natural and holistic exercises, strategies and tips for building your wellness lifestyle from the inside out. Through personal stories and those of other women, expert advice, up-to-date research and timeless principles for living, this book will show you how to nurture your spirit for a lifetime of health, beauty and balance. If you are tired or discouraged by your previous efforts to embrace a healthy lifestyle, I ask you to consider a different approach, to reframe your whole notion about losing weight, exercising, eating well and caring for yourself. When we build a foundation for health grounded in our center—with what comes naturally to us—wellness becomes less of a challenge and more of a lifetime practice of discovery and personal empowerment.

a personal awakening

I grew up in a matriarchal family of immigrants from Haiti. My first exposure to holistic medicine came through my grandmother, who has an encyclopedic knowledge of plants and their medicinal uses. As a girl, I watched her grow medicinal plants in her backyard garden along with tomatoes and other vegetables, occasionally helping her plant the seeds.

In Haitian culture, as in America, women give and give of themselves. Growing up, I watched the women in my family give, hurt, give some more, hurt more and suffer in silence. It is not the Haitian way to openly discuss your problems. So I tacitly learned to keep my thoughts and emotions to myself. I silently absorbed the pain of my parents' divorce and the loss of a wholly nurturing environment. By the time I was in high school, I was thoroughly depressed, but graduation and going to college marked an opportunity for my escape.

As I entered graduate school in my early twenties, I began to develop chronic muscle tension in my neck that eventually spread to other parts of my body. But I kept on running. I lost myself in work and a constant need to achieve and prove myself. I impressed people with my ambition and achievements, yet I was never satisfied. There was always something more to do, something to get or be. By my late twenties, I had been in business for three years and enjoying a considerable amount of success planning and implementing health programs and campaigns that reached national audiences. Then, after managing and promoting a women's health conference, I found myself completely burned out. The stress, long hours and lack of sleep had caught up with me. I felt as if I had nothing left to give, as if my life energy had been sapped. I had reached a breaking point that couldn't be ignored.

I took it as a cue to slow down and get real with myself. I was deeply exhausted, but it wasn't just a physical exhaustion; it was spiritual and emotional fatigue with roots stretching far into my past. I had been carrying a lot of "old stuff" with me and needed to let it go. I realized that for the past ten years I had been living a life of tension and resistance. So I embarked on a journey back to myself that included yoga, meditation, psychotherapy, intense journaling, energy medicine, prayer and study of various spiritual philosophies.

Over the course of several painful and confusing months, it became clear that to be whole and well, I needed to do six things. Those six principles are outlined in this book. I had already been working with these principles throughout the years in various forms, but now they took on a more critical importance. The more I worked with these concepts, the more I felt a change happening inside me. I could feel and appreciate the love that was always there, even though it did not present itself in the way that I wanted. Instead of letting my body be the bearer of blame and discontent, I committed myself to letting it serve as a reflection of divine health, love and beauty. As I moved through this healing process, I felt lighter and more open. I could feel tension being released and a new energy and vitality rising from deep inside of me. I really began to feel myself, my essence, my spirit in my body. I was being guided on a path especially designed for me.

During that period of self-reflection, I realized that wellness is a path of transformation, along which we can heal, develop and integrate all aspects of our being. It is a feeling of connectedness, of being truly alive and awake in one's life. Being awake in mind, body, heart and spirit—that is living well.

the six principles

The following principles and accompanying practices have given me a greater sense of connectedness to myself, God and the world. They've also helped me reconnect with my talents and passions, leading me to write this book.

As you read, I know you'll be inspired and excited to start making changes but don't feel pressure to go out and do anything immediately. Simply receive the information with openness first. You will learn tips, techniques and strategies for slowly reclaiming and empowering yourself, dealing with stress, and learning to trust your innate wisdom to make healthy and life-enhancing choices. Through the principles offered in the following pages, I'll challenge you to:

1. **Open Your Mind to Wellness.** Make the mental shift that is essential to inviting wellness into your life. By aligning your thoughts with your highest intentions, you'll start to create space in your mind and your life for positive, lasting change.

2. **Find Your Balance.** Prioritize your life and keep stress at bay so that you can direct your energy toward people and activities that nourish and uplift you.

3. **Feed Your Spirit.** Enrich yourself through practices and rituals that build your connection to yourself, God and the world so you can enjoy a life of health, purpose and balance.

4. **Open Your Heart.** Balance your emotions and live from the heart by following your passions, learning to forgive, practicing gratitude and giving back.

5. **Honor Your Body.** Use mindfulness to listen to your body, eat wisely and find new joy in exercise and physical activity.

6. **Live in Beauty.** Honor the beauty in yourself and the world as you apply and integrate the principles of wellness into your life.

You'll discover that each day offers opportunities to apply these principles. That's the exciting part! True wellness is a lifelong process, which means every day is a new opportunity to learn, grow and honor the vision and values that we've set for ourselves. Personally, I am still working with these principles. I believe they are seeds, much like the ones that I planted for my grandmother years ago. They are still growing in me. My hope is that you'll find them as helpful on your own journey.

redefining our journey

Although we each have a unique path, we also have a collective path. Women all across the country are hearing that call, opting to simplify their lives, realizing that there has to be a better way to live without being in a constant state of stress, anxiety and denial of our true selves. As such, we are in the midst of a new movement, a movement toward conscious, whole and balanced living. There is no better time to start or redefine our journey than right now. As we individually work toward healing and wholeness, the wisdom, light and love that we gain can not only transform ourselves but also our entire world.

As a woman brings balance to her life physically, emotionally, and spiritually, she fertilizes and replenishes the soil out of which future generations of women grow.

—JANET MACCARO

Wherever you are on the path to living well, you'll find a rich menu of options in the upcoming pages to support you on your journey. Be gentle with yourself and try not to fill yourself up all at once. You can move slowly from one principle to the next, or you can take the à la carte approach, sampling and using only what works for you. The key is to explore and find the practices that speak to you and fit into your life. Set realistic goals for yourself and seek support along the way. Celebrate your successes and find comfort in knowing that your efforts today are leading to a more whole and evolved you.

Let the journey begin!

principle one

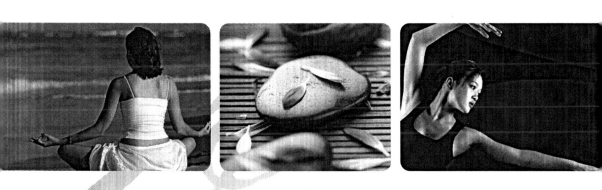

open your mind to wellness

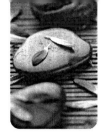

You've heard it before: think positive thoughts for positive health. It sounds too easy, but this simple truth could save your life. Just as cells are the building blocks of our physical bodies, a positive, life-affirming outlook is the foundation of wellness. Positive thinking isn't a cure-all, but it makes a big difference. When we think positively, we move positive energy through our bodies. We affirm our lives, and our cells love that.

Now, you might be skeptical, but there is mounting medical evidence that people who think positively are least likely to be sick or stressed, more likely to recover from a major illness, and more likely to age gracefully. In recent years, medical science has begun to catch up to the time-honored wisdom of ancient healers who understood that we are intricately unified systems consisting of mind, body, heart and spirit. As a woman who loves yoga and can vouch for how it has changed my life, I have incredible respect for the yogis who understood thousands of years ago that manipulating the body with yoga poses stimulates biochemical changes that not only improve health but also alter the practitioner's point of view. Similarly, for every thought there is a physical reaction—a release into the bloodstream of biochemicals called neurotransmitters that carry emotional messages between the brain and body. For example, positive, uplifting thoughts and emotions are accompanied by endorphins, "feel-good" chemicals that elevate mood and create a sense of wellbeing. On the other hand, anxious and fear-based thoughts trigger stress hormones that weaken the immune system and sap our energy and vitality.

In energy medicine, it is believed that all human beings are comprised of energy, which draws from a basic principle in physics that all matter—everything in the universe, not just humans—is comprised of energy, a unifying element. Our cells are always working and consequently vibrating with energy. That energy radiates out, creating an energy field around cells, organs (which are systems of specialized cells) and the entire body. Our energy is affected by what is happening internally and in our environment, including the presence of other energetic bodies (objects or people). Our thoughts, emotions and actions all carry an energy or vibration. We know this instinctively. It's the difference between the person who always has something bad to say and the person who can cheer you up, no matter what is going on. If we know that the way others speak to us can affect us deeply, even changing the mood and atmosphere around us, then imagine the power that positive, affirmative thoughts—high frequency thinking— can have on our health!

Since the 1970s, Dr. Carl Simonton, an internationally known oncologist, and Stephanie Matthews-Simonton, a psychologist, have helped hundreds of patients recover from cancer with the help of visualization. The Simontons developed the visualization program after noticing that patients who had a greater will to live were more likely to return to good health. This was true even for patients in advanced stages of cancer. In another study conducted at Yale University, researchers found that people with an optimistic outlook lived seven and a half years longer than their more gloomy counterparts, their tendency toward positive thinking exerted more of an influence than blood pressure and cholesterol levels. Yet another study of mothers caring for chronically and severely ill children revealed that the extreme stress these otherwise healthy women suffered from caused signs of early aging. The researchers found that stress damages telomeres, the part of DNA in cells that controls aging. Telomeres thin naturally as we grow older, but the telomeres in the blood cells of these mothers were thinning prematurely—*by at least ten years*. But here's the kicker: *the mothers who had a more positive attitude about life did not suffer the same cell damage.*

We have much to learn about how to maintain our health, but one thing is clear: our thoughts have a powerful influence on our overall wellbeing. Thoughts can either hinder or facilitate our path to wellness. They can open or close the door to a myriad of possibilities, opportunities and miracles.

Later in this chapter, you'll complete an exercise that will help you use the power of visualization and affirmative thinking to create a vision of wellness for yourself. Since what we create and envision in our minds can take shape in our bodies and the world around us, this method of opening your mind is a crucial step toward living a life of wellness.

clear your path to positive thinking

I wish I could say that it is easy to just change your mind, to start thinking positively. The reality is that many of us can't imagine, think or speak well of ourselves because of long-held beliefs, often formed when we are young. On top of that, there are stressors and setbacks that make it a challenge to stay on the sunny side. But our thoughts are like flowers—they have to be planted in healthy soil to bloom. Our beliefs are the soil in the gardens of our minds. They shape our thoughts, which are watered by personal experiences and outside influences. Messages we receive from our parents, culture, schooling, friends, lovers, preachers, employers and even strangers leave imprints that affect our current thoughts, emotions and actions. Fortunately, the more awareness we have about why we think the way we do, the more empowered we are to build a new foundation for healthier ways of thinking and being.

Here are four ways to clear your path to a healthy mind and body:

1. *Challenge external messages.* In our age of information, we are constantly bombarded by messages from television, radio, the internet and even our cell phones. The messages flood our consciousness, competing for our time, money and interest. They lure and entice us with ideas of what we *must* know, get, do or be. Inherent in many of the messages is the notion that we are lacking or missing something. The tragedy is that we often believe the ads, which more often than not reinforce messages that we received early in life. The effect of these messages can be imprinted deep in our minds and unconsciously influence how we think, feel and speak to ourselves. As a result, too many women and girls have come to accept that love, health, beauty and wellness lie outside of ourselves, virtues to be had only when we lose weight, have surgery, or find the right product or man.

The almost nonstop messages from the media of what a perfect or attractive body should look like often feeds our feelings of inadequacy. Many women believe deep down that they are unworthy, unattractive and unlikely to ever experience the wellspring of vitality and radiance that lies inside each of us. When we focus on the discontent that we have with our bodies, weight or looks, those thoughts and feelings grow. One negative thought leads to another, creating a negative mindset or frame of mind about ourselves. Imagine the signals that our body receives when we consciously and/or unknowingly dislike ourselves, identify with illness or weakness and/or focus on our faults. When we diminish and devalue ourselves, we are like a boat floating against a river of health and wholeness. When we think in small and limiting ways, we turn down the *rasa*, the juice of life that we were gifted with at birth. That juice is a loving energy, a flow that we can intentionally choose to live in regardless of what others may have to say.

I know, it's easier said than done. But that's why this is a practice. The more we strive to live a conscious lifestyle, the better we'll get at it. It all begins with a conscious decision to look deep within, to draw on the wisdom of your spirit, to design your life and path to wellness from the inside out. In your quest for wellness, you must be willing to tune out the messages that distort the truth and tune in to your inner strength and resources. This is important because so many of us have internalized other people's views and opinions, all the while suppressing and denying our own wisdom, beauty and power. Take a few minutes to begin this process by answering the following questions in your journal:

- What are your core beliefs about yourself? Where did they originate?

- Have the messages from influential people in your life been life-affirming? Confusing? Limiting? Based in fear? Are they useful to you today, or are they holding you down?

- What lessons and strengths (like resiliency or independence) have you gained from your upbringing and past experiences, including negative ones? How can use them on your path to wellness?

- What do you believe about health, illness and challenging life events? Do you believe that you're destined to become ill or inherit a disease?

- How do you feel about aging?

- Do you believe that you are worthy, deserving and capable of living the best and healthiest life possible for yourself?

- What do you believe about the purpose and meaning of your life? Are your current thoughts, attitudes and actions in line with your beliefs about your life?

By rooting out or at least exposing the origins of thoughts that block our ability to live optimally, we are creating space for that whole and complete woman inside each of us to find freedom to express herself and say "YES!" to life. And isn't that what this is all about? To live with heart by saying "yes" to life, love, health, peace, passion and joy.

2. Remember who you are. Be warned that as you change your thoughts and your life, your ego, which is attached to the opinions of others, will put up a fight. It feeds off of thoughts of vulnerability and clouds our ability to see the truth.

We are born into a natural state of wholeness and closeness to Source. Our spirits shine through us freely. We have a light in our eyes. It is the same light that grabs you while standing impatiently in line at the grocery store and makes you laugh with the baby in the next aisle. That light is waiting to be reclaimed by you. The baby (let's call her Sarah) has a universal connection to everyone. Sarah does not see herself as separate from you, me or anyone else. But as we grow, the ego is formed and shaped by our family, friends and life experiences. To make sense of what has happened to and around us, the mind constructs the ego, which becomes the basis of our identity and sense of self. The ego forms at a very early age and exerts a powerful influence on how we see ourselves and the world. It is a mask we wear to help us navigate relationships, roles, responsibilities and other aspects of life. The formation of the ego in and of itself is not a bad thing—it is a critical stage in our development. By age three, psychologists say that a child has already begun to adjust its behavior to obtain approval of others. Although its best intentions are to protect us, the ego is not always rational and is often built on a foundation of fear, pain and confusion. It is from this shaky foundation that we operate as adults—until we decide to rebuild a healthier foundation for our lives.

To protect us, the ego reinforces thoughts, beliefs and memories that confirm our perceived separateness from Source and from others. The result makes us strong and independent, but it can also create more painful feelings: *I'm alone in this world. I can't trust anyone.* So, over time, Sarah will eventually stop smiling at strangers. Any number of scripts about why she shouldn't smile or say hello might run through her head when she sees someone she doesn't know: *I don't want to be hurt. They won't smile back. We don't smile or speak to strangers. She's different, she's white, black or Latino, etc.*

One day when I was sitting quiet and feeling like a motherless child, which I was, it came to me: that feeling of being part of everything, not separate at all. I knew that if I cut a tree, my arm would bleed.

—SHUG AVERY, IN ALICE WALKER'S *THE COLOR PURPLE*

Sarah, like many of us early on, learns in subtle ways from her parents, peers and society—either by force or simply looking at the world around her—

to see herself as separate and having to fend for herself. Life experiences and events in her young, developing mind will only confirm that perceived reality. Her parents get divorced, for example, and she's left devastated by the event. Her ego has a field day trying to explain what has happened: *I'm alone. I'm not loved. I can't trust anyone. I'm never getting married.* Childhood wounds like divorce leave indelible imprints on us, especially if we aren't guided in a way that facilitates healing and understanding. Our ego is left unchecked to figure things out.

Sarah's story is very much my story and the story of countless other women and men. When we are hurt, either in childhood or as adults, our ego sees these painful events as confirmation that we are vulnerable beings that must always be in protection mode. When we think in this way, we close our hearts and spirits to the fullness and wholeness of who we are. Instead, we live in limits rather than possibilities. But if we believe that we are the offspring of a wonderful, creative and limitless power, then how can we be any different? When we create something, a part of us is in that creation. Likewise, the creative spark of the divine is always within us, and we can use it to design the fullest and healthiest life possible for ourselves.

A woman is the full circle. Within her is the power to create, nurture and transform.

—DIANE MARIECHILD

When we choose to change the thoughts and misperceptions that limit our full expression and potential, we reclaim our birthright. *A Course in Miracles* reminds us that health is our natural state when we rely on God to interpret the meaning and purpose of our lives. When our ego takes over this responsibility, the interpretation is usually based in fear and lack. The *Course* also notes that "health is inner peace." We can't have peace and health if we are in constant conflict with who we are. We have been gifted with minds that have the power to create and bring out the beauty in ourselves and others. But if we believe that health and beauty are out-side of ourselves—that we must get them from others or from a bottle or other substances—then we are in denial of our

our minds and bodies are nurtured with healing and positive thoughts that affirm our truth

true selves. When we can align our thoughts with our deepest desires and prayers to be well, to be whole and find inner peace, we are closer to coming home and living our truth. In the words of John Keats, "Beauty is truth." When we are living our truth, we are beautiful.

Health, peace, love and beauty is in every cell in my body. I am health. I am peace. I am beauty. I am whole. I am well.

—AFFIRMATION FOR WELLNESS

3. Turn wounds into wisdom. Sometimes we have to look back to move forward. Looking back at the past illuminates the present by providing insight into the experiences that shaped our beliefs and our lives up to today.

Understandably, there may be a lot of fear in revisiting painful life experi-ences, but if they are affecting your health and quality of life, it's worth it to take a look back—with an eye toward moving forward without getting stuck in the past or identifying with your wounds and illnesses.

Caroline Myss, Ph.D., medical intuitive and author of *Why People Don't Heal,* observes that people can adopt a "woundology" attitude in which they define themselves by their wounds, not wanting to move beyond them. When our identity is tied to our wounds, Myss says, "we burden and lose our physical and spiritual energy and open ourselves to the risk of illness." And yet pain, illness and adversity can be transformative. It's all in how we choose to view things. We can choose to see wounds and disappointments as permanent road blocks or opportunities for deep insight and change. We can do this exploratory work through journaling, self-help books, personal development seminars, women's support groups and professional therapy. We can do this alone but finding help provides the support we all need when embarking on life-changing experiences.

And the day came when the risk it took to remain tight in the bud was more painful than the risk it took to blossom.

—ANAIS NIN

4. Talk to a professional. Having someone like a spiritual counselor or therapist who is completely devoted to listening to you objectively and without judgment can be very healing. Psychotherapy can help you make breakthroughs you may not be able to achieve on your own. It has helped me to delve deeper into my own life experiences in a way I couldn't have by myself. It's not just about exploring the past but gaining insight and inner strength to face challenges today and tomorrow. There is still some lingering stigma about psychotherapy, though most of it appears to be gone, thank heavens! Many of us run to the doctor when we have a physical ache—why not when we need help with the most fundamental aspects of our being? A good therapist understands how to help clients rediscover and live from their core selves.

We don't have to suffer or figure things out on our own. Accepting that we need help to heal ourselves is part of transcending the ego-fueled misperception that we are alone. "If we are willing to do the mental work, almost anything can be healed," said Louise Hay, author of *You Can Heal Your Life.* Hay completely healed herself of cancer in six months through a program of affirmations, visualizations, nutritional cleansings and psychotherapy.

If you choose to work with a therapist, do your research. Find out what school of thought the therapist comes from and the type of training the therapist has received. Ask questions. I personally needed someone who used body-centered approaches and actively sought out a core energetics psychotherapist who uses the body and physical movement to help clients access, feel and release emotions. Blocked emotions can be toxic, lodging themselves in our muscles and triggering "unexplainable" aches and physical symptoms.

You should interview a few therapists to find the right fit. It may take a few sessions to figure out. If it is not the right fit, find another therapist that you are comfortable with, but don't give up. We all need someone to speak to openly and without judgment. Many of the people we think we can turn to have their own issues and enough to fully listen and really *hear* what we have to say. The reality is that our attention span is often too short—an effect of our fast-paced, multitasked world. People can also be incredibly uncomfortable with silence. And sometimes all we need is someone to listen without interjecting and filling the silence with empty words.

Recently, while attending a workshop led by an Israeli storyteller, I was reminded of the power of silence and how uncomfortable it can be. During the session—filled with women of various ages and ethnicities—each of us was asked to share a story about love from our lives. We were all given a set time to share our story. If we finished before the allotted time, we were to just sit there and not say anything. We did this several times, each time with someone else and eventually in groups of four. The first few times were awkward, staring at a stranger, not saying a word after she had shared an intimate part of her life. Naturally, we broke the "sit in silence rule," choosing instead to make jokes about how uncomfortable it was to not say anything. By the end of the day, we had all gotten much better at it and could appreciate the value of just sitting in silence, honoring each others' stories. There is a real art to listening and asking the right questions. A good therapist or counselor has those skills and can help lead you to healing and resolution.

find your peace of mind

How would you describe your current outlook on life? Are you seeing the glass as half full or half empty? When something goes wrong, can you see the light at the end of the tunnel, the lesson in the challenge and the hope in the despair? An important first step toward reframing our thoughts is observing how we think in a nonjudgmental way. It's important that we don't label our thoughts and feelings as "bad." They are what they are. A more effective approach is to ask yourself whether your thoughts are working toward your higher good. If they **are** not, it's time to try something new. Remember, your thoughts may be grounded in fear or a period of time in your life that has long since passed.

Below are solutions for combating five common modes of thinking that can limit your perception of yourself and your life. Reframing the way you look at life and its challenges is an essential step toward achieving health and peace of mind. These tips will help you develop healthier patterns of thinking that lay the foundation for an optimistic outlook and mindset.

- *Put an end to perfectionism.* We are inundated with ideals of what women *should* look like. Define health and beauty for yourself. Know that comparing yourself to others doesn't serve you. Instead, remember the beauty and strength you carry inside. Set realistic goals and use yourself as the barometer for progress and success. See principle 2 for more on perfectionism.

- *Banish catastrophic thinking.* Have you had a setback with your weight loss goals? Maybe you or a loved one has recently been diagnosed with a chronic health condition. These types of situations can be painful but don't have to be the end of the world. Choose to see the opportunity in the challenge. Ask yourself: Is there a lesson here for me? How can I enjoy the present moment? Count your blessings. Choose to see the positive instead of just the negative, such as the happy memories you have of someone who is gravely ill or has passed away.

- *Let go of your attachment to results and things.* We live in a results-driven society, programmed to seek the fruits of our labor. This in and of itself isn't a bad thing, but it orients us toward always looking for something in return. When we don't achieve the success or recognition we'd hoped for, disappointment and disillusionment can set in. Try doing something simply for the love of it, or because it brings you fulfillment or helps someone else. So many times, we embark on a new diet or exercise plan because we want to look nice in time for a big event or to impress others. But what about taking care of ourselves simply out of love and respect for the body and life we have been given?

Take note of what you really need to live well. Do you really need the expensive car, big house, all those clothes? Over our lifetime we accumulate more and more things, and some are necessary to enhance, beautify and simplify our lives. But our stuff can become a part of the mask we create to hide our insecurities from ourselves and the world. Different things have different meaning to different people. Only you know. But a good place to start is by asking yourself if your possessions define who you are.

• **Stop worrying.** Constructive worrying helps us prepare for the future. We purchase health insurance in case we need medical care, and we save for a rainy day. With constructive worrying, concern for the future is followed by healthy, constructive action. But what about times when little or nothing can be done about the past or future, or when we jump to conclusions because we lack information? Destructive worrying is a repetitive pattern of anxious or fearful thinking with no resolution. It keeps us stuck in a state of fear and inaction. Instead of being swept away by your worries, try scheduling a time to worry. Write down your thoughts, doubts and fears

> *I concentrate on a solution instead of a problem. By doing this, I am constantly working toward a goal—which is positive, instead of constantly focusing on the problem, which is negative.*
>
> —KESHA, AGE 35

and then determine what you can do about them. Acknowledging your worries in this way can stop the repetitive thoughts about them. Move toward the resolution of the ones you can take action on. The longer you remain in a state of inaction, the more you will worry. If the situation is beyond your control, move toward acceptance. Define for yourself what acceptance of the situation will look and feel like to you. When you find yourself worrying, tell yourself to stop or find another activity like meditation, exercise or deep breathing to shift your attention from your worrying thoughts. We may not be able to control the future, but research shows that we can do something right now that could help: think positively.

- **Be open to change.** Do you feel stuck? Are you unable to lose weight or make life-enhancing changes? Changing your perspective and approach can be the real solution to getting "unstuck." Trying to change your behavior without addressing the underlying issues that get in the way of real, sustainable change is like trying to go up on a down escalator. I often get frustrated by ads for weight loss products promising to help you lose weight without making any lifestyle changes. The path of least resistance isn't always the best path, and it's rarely the most effective. We learn and grow so much more when we challenge and stretch ourselves.

    Is it time to apply a different brushstroke to your life? Choose new colors, materials and possibilities for yourself. When you resist change or ignore your inner voice, conflict and unease will arise. In order to evolve into the person you were intended to be, you must extend and reach beyond what you see, know and experience. The more you reflect on your life experiences and growth, the more love you'll have for yourself. You'll develop a greater appreciation for your ability to adjust, adapt and accept.

Treasured ancient masterpieces go through a restoration process to repair cracks, dullness and blemishes. You can do the same for your life.

picture yourself well

Pictures are powerful motivators. It's why magazines and newspapers are filled with eye-catching photos—sometimes photos say more than words ever could. Pictures can go past our rational minds and touch us at our core, even if we don't consciously agree with the message. This is why it's so important to feed our minds with positive images that support what we want to bring into our lives.

When used with powerful techniques, such as visualization and meditation, positive thinking can break down the negative thought patterns that hold us back from living in health, beauty and balance.

A perfect example of the power of pictures was demonstrated when Harvard researchers showed a group of college students a video clip of Mother Teresa helping poor people on the streets of Calcutta. Blood tests taken before and after viewing the footage revealed that the students' immune systems were boosted as a result of watching the clips. Even the immune systems of those students who had a cynical response to the film or stated that they did not admire Mother Teresa were strengthened.

Visualization can be a fun and affirmative way to not only open your mind to new possibilities but also generate the positive energy you need to stay motivated as you build or refine your overall wellness practice and work toward specific goals, such as losing weight or becoming more physically active. Charlotte Manning, a minister and motivational speaker, fills her visualizations with vivid and colorful details. The enthusiasm she expresses as she speaks about her vision is infectious, "As I enter my dream house, I am greeted by four steps: the first says 'spirit', the second 'mind', the third 'body'. The last step says 'this is the house that God created'. As I enter the home I say to myself, 'I've connected.'" To continually remind herself of this larger vision for her life, Charlotte created a vision board (discussed below) and keeps a picture of it on her cell phone. She also paints her toes red. Whenever she looks at her toes, she has a visual reminder of the ultimate goal of walking on those steps and entering the home and life of her dreams.

The future belongs to those who believe in the beauty of their dreams.

—ELEANOR ROOSEVELT

Are you ready to create the picture of a well you, living with mind, body, heart and spirit in total harmony? The following four-step process will help you use the combined power of visualization and affirmation to develop your unique picture of wellness. It is important that the picture reflects your personal goals and not what others might think you should do or be. Be realistic, but don't limit yourself either. Your picture may change once you get to the end of the book, but it is important that you begin to set the intention and create the vision for your life right now. You will want to return to this exercise once you complete the book and during or after major life changes or transitions.

Before you begin, find a quiet place where you will not be interrupted. Calm your mind and relax your body by closing your eyes and tuning in to your breath for a few minutes. Focusing on your breath will help center you. Take a few deep breaths or simply place your hands on your belly and observe the movement. Give yourself permission to be completely present in the moment as you complete each step.

1. Define wellness for yourself. Wellness is a unique expression of our physical conditions and capabilities, life experiences, emotional and spiritual needs, passions and goals. Wellness for me might be running a marathon with only a minimal amount of pain in my knees and legs, whereas your picture of wellness might be speaking or dancing in public, freely expressing who you are without fear. Or it might be simply coming to terms with a chronic illness or disability, where you are maintaining the best quality of life possible for yourself and doing what you love. It could be feeling energetic and vibrant by taking great care of yourself, keeping stress at bay, eating more fruits and vegetables or staying physically active. There are so many ways that we can be pictures of wellness.

To create the picture, ask yourself the following questions:

- What is wellness to me?

- What will wellness feel like? How might it be expressed in my mind, body, heart and spirit?

  Mind—I am thinking positively, fearlessly.

  Body—I have more energy than ever before; I am listening to my body.

  Heart—I am doing what I am passionate about; I am in touch with my emotions.

  Spirit—My life has meaning and purpose; I feel loved and connected to myself, God, family and community.

- What do I need to do to be well? What makes me feel whole and centered?

- What would the "well me" look like? What would I be doing?

The responses provided under the second bullet above are just examples. Answer these questions according to your own needs, desires and capabilities. Allow yourself freedom to dream and be open to new possibilities. Don't let fear or past failure at attempts to improve your health limit your vision. You should also refrain from thinking about what you need to do to achieve your vision right now. The remaining principles provide a toolkit of ideas, resources and solutions for you to consider as you move into the action phase of creating your wellness lifestyle. At this point, you are simply creating the picture. Tell yourself: *I am creating a new vision for my life with a new foundation grounded in love. I am releasing the thoughts, beliefs and attitudes that no longer serve me. I am open to this journey of self-discovery.* Several years ago, I worked for a company that coached women to do extraordinary things, such as walking sixty miles in three days to raise money and awareness about breast cancer. The company's motto was "I'm possible." Believe that you—the healthy, whole, balanced and complete you—is possible.

2. Set your intentions. The following step is inspired by the practice of yoga nidra (yogic sleep), in which a *sankalpa*, resolve about something you deeply wish to see in your life, is brought into awareness on two levels: verbally and visually. On the verbal level, you develop a simple statement or affirmation that reflects your deepest desire. In this case, your sankalpa might be "I am healthy and whole," or "I am full of energy, peace and love."

For me, "I am well" says it all. It speaks to my desire to be healthy at all levels of my being, at peace in God's love and fully expressing my gifts and purpose. Your sankalpa should be simple and rooted in your desire to experience wellness. It should speak to you and move you at the deepest level of your being. You should be able to associate a feeling with your sankalpa. For example, "I am well" conjures up feelings of completeness and wholeness for me. Use the answers to the questions in step 1 to help you develop your sankalpa or resolve. If you are having difficulty formulating your sankalpa, set an intention to be open to discovering your deepest desire. Be patient and open to the idea that it may reveal itself through your dreams, meditation, journaling and other people.

3. Formulate and work with your mental picture. The next step is to formulate a mental image of yourself doing or experiencing your sankalpa. The image should say it all. Recall the examples in step 1 of completing a marathon, dancing in public or adjusting to a chronic condition. Your image should encapsulate all the feelings and desires you associate with your sankalpa. Throughout the day or whenever you meditate, repeat your sankalpa to yourself and/or call up the mental picture of your sankalpa. Because meditation brings you to a calm and receptive state where you can see yourself in a new light, it is a useful tool for transcending the thoughts, fears and doubts that prevent us from realizing our wellness goals.

Practice this visualization regularly. Anytime you have a few moments to close your eyes and imagine your picture will help—before you get out of bed in the morning or while soaking in the tub, for instance. The picture may seem fuzzy at first, but practice will sharpen the image. Over time, you'll find that calling up your mental picture will create a sense of calm and connectedness that shifts your perspective. Try doing this when stressed and see what happens.

A great way to enhance your visualization experience is to use a guided visualization or yoga nidra tape, CD or mp3. Working with an audio recording will provide additional structure and guidance in the early stages of your visualization. You may also want to make a tape of yourself stating and describing your affirmations. Hearing our own voices can have an incredible effect on our subconscious minds. There is no other voice like your own. It is a unique combination of your breath, emotion, and internal vibrations. My former voice coach, Mary Naden, describes the voice as the way we release ourselves into the world. Her approach to the voice isn't to train people to "speak properly" but to find their true voice, which may have been influenced and hindered by upbringing, environment, physical and psychological stress. By vocalizing your sankalpa and affirmations, you are "putting them out into the universe." That's a powerful step toward creating the beautiful and healthy life you want and deserve.

4. Face your inner critic. If you've developed your sankalpa but feel some resistance, acknowledge it. Flush out all the barriers that may prevent you from achieving your sankalpa. Let's say you want to lose weight but think you can't. Ask yourself, *Where are these thoughts coming from? Is my past experience of not losing weight influencing my ability to see myself in a new way? What will I do differently this time around?* A lot of your ability to make healthy lifestyle changes will depend on your relationship with your body and how you view the behavioral changes you need to make. If you have feelings of resentment, guilt or shame toward your body, take a moment and think about when and where these feelings started. More often than not, they probably didn't start with you. It was probably something you heard or saw that made you start thinking your body wasn't beautiful enough. They were not your original thoughts, but you absorbed them and they have become a part of you, until now. If instead you decide to lose weight out of love for your body and life, your whole approach will be different. It won't be a battle against your body, but a natural part of living a healthy lifestyle. (Please refer to the Love Your Body section in principle 5 for more on this topic.)

Reframing your thoughts into positive, affirmative statements that honor who you are will move you much closer to your goal than self-critical thoughts. So instead of "I'll never lose this extra weight," try "I am committed to seeing and being a healthier me." Take note of the limiting thoughts and beliefs that might be holding you back. For every pessimistic thought, develop an affirmation to counter it. But don't dwell too much on the negative. Let your inner critic have her say, then move on.

5. Map your treasure. In this step you will create a treasure map or vision board. You'll need at least an hour for this practice. Gather a few magazines, scissors, tape or glue and a large poster board. Flip through the pages of the magazines, cutting out pictures and words that capture the feelings and activities associated with your sankalpa. Once you have pictures representing your key goals, create a collage by pasting or taping them onto the poster board in an arrangement that works for you. Once you've completed your vision board, post it somewhere you'll be able to see it daily. As you see the photos, even if you're not paying attention, they will be imprinted on your subconscious mind. If you don't want your treasure map to be seen by others, place it in a drawer or book that you open often. You can also create a smaller version within your journal or appointment book. Your vision board is an affirmative representation of your deepest desires and having someone laugh, criticize or project other negative energy toward your goals counters what you are trying to do. Treasure and honor the entire process.

principle two

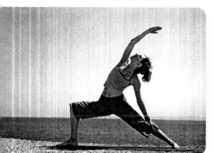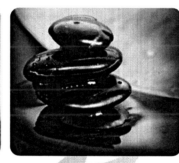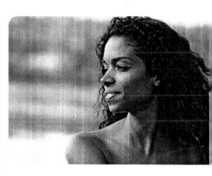

find your balance

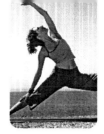

Stress

Stress is eating away at our energy, zest and vitality. Far too many women are drained by daily living to actually live. We're "too tired" to exercise or "too busy" to set aside time for ourselves. We have become so focused on getting things done and resolving problems that our lives feel like an endless stream of tasks and challenges. More women than ever are feeling the pressure to excel both at home and at work. We are mothers, wives, caregivers, employees and businesswomen. We often overextend ourselves and feel pulled in many directions. While we may enjoy the various roles that enrich our lives, the stress of wearing multiple hats—and the feeling that we're unable to take any of them off—places many women in an emotional and physical danger zone.

According to the American Institute of Stress, stress is the nation's number one health problem. Somewhere between 60 percent and 90 percent of all physician visits are for stress-related complaints. The frenzied pace of modern living leaves little time for nurturing the vital dimensions of life that keep us going every day.

As the major barrier to living well today, we cannot fully embark on our journey to wellness without addressing stress and its effect on our lives. Until we confront the stressors that are blocking our experience of health and wholeness, we are just dipping our toe in the water when we really want to swim.

stress effects: mind, body, heart and spirit

Stress can numb us out of feeling and experiencing the present. Over time, the stress of our high-speed lives can leave us feeling fractured, like we've divided or even lost parts of ourselves. It's that sense of "I feel like I'm all over the place" that many women express. Out of tune with ourselves and the desires of our hearts, we make choices reflective of others' demands and expectations instead of our values and priorities.

Tension is who you think you should be.
Relaxation is who you are.

—CHINESE PROVERB

Stress can affect our ability to sleep, trigger headaches and muscular tension, disrupt our digestive and immune systems, diminish our sex drive and contribute to premature aging. It can reduce our ability to focus, decrease productivity, lead to depression and contribute to a general sense of powerlessness and anxiety.

While stress is unavoidable, it is manageable. This is an idea that is hard for many of us to accept, especially if we are the primary decision makers at home or lack social support and assistance. I've known women to get resentful and even angry when I've suggested taking small steps to manage stress, such as a five-minute walk in one instance. "When you're taking care of the family and working long hours, how can you do that?" a woman I care deeply about snapped back at me. I felt sad that although she was clearly having medical problems as a result of her stress, she didn't value herself enough to start taking better care of herself.

To deal with stress, many women turn to food, smoking and other unhealthy behaviors. According to a recent survey conducted by the American Psychological Association in partnership with iVillage.com and the National Women's Health Resource Center, women are more likely to engage in comfort eating due to stress. Emotional eating can result in obesity, which in turn raises the risk of developing heart disease, diabetes and a host of other health problems. Additionally, women who work long hours are more likely to consume caffeine and high-fat and high-sugar snacks. They are also more likely to smoke and to forego exercise.

In my lifestyle coaching program, emotional eating was a frequent contributor to weight problems among participants. Not surprisingly, more than half of the women who joined the program were either borderline or at high-risk for developing depression and stress-related complications. Women are twice as likely as men to suffer from depression—a serious and often overlooked obstacle to wellness.

stress and our hearts

Chronic stress can pose a serious risk to our hearts. While our bodies are capable of withstanding a considerable amount of stress, prolonged stress can chip away at us and create conditions ripe for a heart attack.

- When under stress, many women often engage in unhealthy behaviors (such as overeating and smoking) that raise their risk of heart disease.

- Overtime, stress can lower estrogen levels, which has been linked to heart disease — the number one killer of women.

- Depression has been linked to heart rhythm abnormalities and can double the risk of developing heart disease.

- Stress increases blood pressure and homocysteine—a dietary byproduct of animal protein. Elevated levels of homocysteine damages arteries, making it easier for cholesterol deposits to form in artery walls.

- Stress constricts arteries and muscles, encourages irregular heart rhythms and increases blood clotting.

Stress affects our weight in another way as well. We are wired to deal with stress through the "fight or flight" response. If we sense danger, our bodies immediately release hormones to aid in either physically fighting the stressor or escaping it. This response explains why, when faced with a threat, we suddenly experience extraordinary physical strength and energy to protect ourselves or loved ones. Thankfully, most of us aren't faced with these types of threats on a daily basis. The downside is that our brains do not differentiate between the type of stress and the response it elicits. So the daily stresses we face will still result in the release of cortisol, a stress hormone that increases appetite. The idea is that since we are either going to fight or fly, we are going to need more food for energy. Yet our responses to most of our stressors are not physical, so we are not burning off the extra weight that our bodies have stored up.

recognize the symptoms of stress

We all respond to stress differently. What may be stressful for one person may be a welcome source of change for another. Yet we often underestimate the impact that stress has on our lives. We tell ourselves that we can handle things (often on our own), but at what cost? Major life events such as divorce or the death of a spouse or family member or a few small yet stressful events occurring within a relatively short period of time, can affect our ability to adjust to change in healthy ways. Even positive events such as getting married, having a baby or taking on a promotion can be stressful. Adjusting to a new life or set of demands on our time and attention can test and tax our ability to adapt.

Below is a list of common symptoms of stress. Your doctor can help you determine whether the following symptoms may be signs of stress or another condition or illness:

- Insomnia
- Headaches
- Backaches
- Muscular tension
- High blood pressure
- Irregular menstrual periods
- Chest pains
- Shortness of breath
- Skin blemishes, acne or cold sores
- Fatigue

- Poor memory

- Overeating

- Difficulty concentrating

- Moodiness or depression

- Feelings of dissatisfaction and unhappiness

simplify your life to restore balance and alleviate stress

Often, it is our response to stress that knocks us off balance. Fortunately, by limiting and effectively coping with stress, we can minimize its emotional and physical toll on our lives. The two-step plan below will help you grab a hold of stress and begin to create the life of wellness that you envision. Step 1 will help you simplify your life by focusing on what really matters. The second step, *Learn to Relax,* includes a variety of simple, holistic ways to relax and alleviate stress.

STEP 1: SIMPLIFY YOUR LIFE
prioritize your life

While stress is inevitable, the good news is that you can reduce and at times completely eliminate certain stressors by prioritizing your life. Prioritizing tasks and responsibilities and delegating and eliminating non-essential activities will free up time to enjoy more of life.

Consider how you would ideally like to spend your time. What's standing in the way? Are there certain tasks or responsibilities preventing you from doing what you enjoy? Place a premium on your time and your life. Make a list of the things that you *have* to do on a daily or weekly basis. Are these things absolutely necessary? Are you afraid to say no and taking on projects even though you're already spread thin or pressed for time? Are there tasks that you can delegate to someone else? In my business, I struggled with what I could afford to hire people to do, so I did a lot myself. But I realized very early that although it was an additional expense, I had to hire an accountant. I didn't have the time, expertise or desire to handle this part of the business on my own.

As you think about the questions above, consider whether there are new or alternative methods you can employ to save time and reduce the burden of completing certain tasks. Be creative. Don't allow excuses to get in the way of making changes. You may have to make some concessions, but consider all your options and the benefits you'll reap from the extra time you'll gain.

Two-Step Plan to Restore Balance and Alleviate Stress

Step 1: Simplify Your Life

- Prioritize your life.
- Commit to self care and compassion.
- End the juggling act.
- Let superwoman fly.

Step 2: Learn to Relax

- Breathe deeply.
- Move your body.
- Call upon friends and family.
- Smell the roses.
- Let the Music Play.

Be realistic about balance and life. Life is dynamic, yet our concept of balance is that it's a state we're always in—or, at least, that we're supposed to be in. It would be nice if that were true, but approaching life in such a way can stress you out! Accept that there will be times when certain areas of your life will take precedence over others. I like the philosophy that we can have it all, just not all at the same time. A major deadline at work may require you to spend more time working than usual. A child or loved one may fall sick and you may have to direct more of your energy and time toward helping him heal.

Life is what happens to you while you are busy making other plans.

—JOHN LENNON

commit to self-care and compassion

Self-care should be at the top of your list of priorities. Take self-care seriously by scheduling "me time" in your calendar or adding it to your to-do list. Commit to giving yourself a minimum of thirty minutes each day to connect with yourself through meditation, yoga, journaling, prayer or just sitting in silence. Regularly affirming yourself, your purpose and divine presence in your life will inspire a sense of gratitude and connectedness to your daily life and work. It can also help reframe your responsibilities into acts of devotion, love and service to others.

Our natural impulse to care for others can be a major challenge when balancing priorities. While a large part of what gives meaning to our lives is service to others, it should not be at the expense of oneself. A number of studies on caregiver burden have shown that caregivers, usually women, often become sick themselves during or soon after caring for sick loved ones. As a graduate student, I worked at the American Cancer Society studying this very issue. Our natural inclination is to care and nurture, yet we often forget to give ourselves the same loving attention. When we make self-care a priority, the people and world around us benefit. We have more energy, love and patience to share—and that's a win-win for everyone involved.

Create and honor your boundaries. Friends and family will be more likely to take your commitment to self-care seriously if you do. If guilt or feelings of selfishness creep up, remind yourself that self-care is about your health and livelihood. When we take our life into perspective, our priorities often change. It should not have to take a major health crisis for us to slow down and realize what matters most. Our lives do indeed depend on how well we take care of ourselves. If we don't put ourselves first, who else will?

Here are a few ideas for pampering and nurturing yourself that you can start using today:

- *Retreat*. Steal away each day for a minimum of thirty minutes for "me time." If you have children, hire a babysitter or make a pact with a friend to watch each other's children when you need to retreat for an hour or two.

- *Take Your Lunch Break.* Instead of sitting in front of your desk during lunch, eat at a park or near a lake. Build in some time to take a short walk before or after your meal.

- *Take a Weekly Bath.* Fill your tub with warm water and add a few drops of your favorite essential oils (see Smell the Roses section later in this chapter).

end the juggling act

It's hard to imagine not multitasking with all that we have to do these days. Multitasking has become our method to deal with the madness. But trying to juggle so many balls at one time increases stress and anxiety and makes us irritable. New research in the area of multitasking has shown that while some multitasking can be beneficial, it may actually decrease productivity and performance. The more tasks an individual juggles, the less productive she becomes. When we juggle several tasks at once, it takes longer to complete each individual task than if we focused on completing them one at a time. When we stop juggling, we become more mindful and present in everyday tasks and encounters. This is a simple and radical shift in consciousness that can dramatically change our lives.

> *I take time away from my daily routine at least twice a month to spend time with friends or get a massage. Occasionally, I attend women's spiritual retreats mainly to fellowship with other women for a period of time away from my husband, kids and job. I've learned that I am not alone in the challenges that I face. There are so many women out there struggling with the same issues.*
>
> .—KARLA, AGE 37

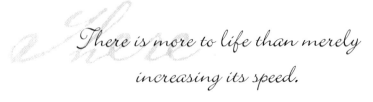

There is more to life than merely increasing its speed.

—GANDHI

As a recovering workaholic, the feeling that I had no time to process things, was a major impetus for slowing down. It felt as if I was living in a twilight zone where every day blended into the next, with no separation, no lines, just one day of work after work after work. There was always one more thing I needed to get done before I got to sleep, eat or head for a meeting. There will always be something else that has to get done. We just have to accept that some things have to wait and that we simply can't do everything at one time. Life coach and best-selling author Cheryl Richardson urges women to give up the juggling act and let some balls drop. "Stop trying to be a star and stop trying to do everything," Richardson says.

let superwoman fly

In the television show *Desperate Housewives*, Marcia Cross plays the role of Bree Van De Kamp, a stay-at-home mom who is the epitome of extreme perfectionism. She rarely shows emotion and keeps a "perfect" house, regularly cooking gourmet meals. She neatly puts her feelings aside and picks up the pieces when things fall apart. She is "well-bred" and expects her children to be too. Bree's wayward son shocked her one day by asking her to prepare a real meal instead of "cuisine."

Desperate Housewives was a runaway hit because many women found humor in it and could relate to the insanity of the lives of the main characters. Bree's perfectionism is over the top, but far too many of us have a "Bree" inside of us, always wanting to stay in charge and in control. We want it all: a happy home life, success at work, a great body and material possessions. There is nothing wrong with wanting the best and striving to live our best life. The problem is that we sometimes obsess over it. And it can be hard not to. From an early age, we are bombarded by images of the "ideal" woman. We internalize other people's definition of what it is to be a "good" mother, wife or career woman. We exhaust ourselves trying to keep up with expectations, often unrealistic ones that we have created for ourselves.

When we seek perfection, nothing is ever good enough—including our perceptions of ourselves. Alexandra Stoddard, interior decorator and lifestyle philosopher, states in her book, *The Art of the Possible: The Path From Perfectionism to Balance and Freedom,* that when the "inclination toward perfectionism becomes obsessive, we become driven by our narrow view of what is important." Perfectionism is a form of self-protection used to hide that we are in fact in crisis and lack control, Stoddard explains. Fixating on what happened in the past or what needs to be done in the future takes us away from the present.

Country music superstar Naomi Judd decided to "resign as general manager of the universe" after she was diagnosed with Hepatitis C. She was often bedridden and lacked the energy to pursue her usual perfectionist tendencies. "I could no longer be my old perfectionist, do-it-all self. It wasn't an option—I just did not have the strength. Besides, it was standing in the way of having more fun and pleasure."

The perfect you isn't something you need to create, because God already created it. The perfect you is the love within you.

—MARIANNE WILLIAMSON

For some, it is the escape from reality—perhaps an unloved or unfulfilling reality—that drives perfectionist tendencies. The stress from constantly seeking to be perfect—or hiding the fact that we are not—can harm our health. Paul Hewitt, Ph.D., and Gordon Flett, Ph.D., have studied perfectionism for over twenty years. Their research has shown that perfectionism is associated with depression, anxiety, eating disorders and a host of other mental health problems. According to Hewitt, perfectionism often stems from interpersonal needs, such as the need to be loved or accepted.

The Hewitt and Flett research team identified three types of perfectionists: Self-oriented perfectionists set high standards for themselves; other-oriented perfectionists set unrealistic standards for those around them; and socially imposed perfectionists feel that others, such as family, school or religion, are demanding perfection of them.

Perfectionism not only takes its toll on the perfectionist, but also on those around her. It can cause conflicts and rifts between the perfectionist and her coworkers, friends and family members. The rigid standards of a perfectionist can strain relationships. It can be quite unpleasant to be around someone who constantly nags, never sees the good in anyone's efforts or has impossibly high standards for herself and everyone around her. While we should not settle for less, we should consider whether the high standards that we have set are hurting ourselves and others. It is usually the reaction to not having a standard met that leads the perfectionist to adopt unhealthy behaviors and attitudes. Beating ourselves up over failures and

I've learned to relax and just enjoy life more—not to always take life so seriously. I love to laugh and have a good laugh everyday.
—SYLVIA, AGE 54

mistakes is not a useful exercise. Finding lessons and opportunities for growth in disappointments can help us achieve the excellence we seek in our relationships, work, health and life. Again, it comes down to a healthy, balanced perspective.

In the 1980s, fitness expert Susan Powter's motto was "stop the insanity." The need to be perfect in all we do is driving us crazy. It's time that we stop the insanity. We are not superwomen with superhuman powers. It's time to let super-woman fly. To start, consider the following questions:

- Am I a perfectionist? If yes, why? What is driving my perfectionist behavior?

- Are the standards, expectations and goals I have set for myself reason-able? Are they realistic? What are these standards costing me? Is it worth it?

- What do I obsess about? What absolutely has to be done "my way or the highway?"

- If I let go of my perfectionist tendencies, will my life be simpler? Less stressful?

If you're a perfectionist, ask a friend or a counselor to help you work through your perfectionist behaviors. An objective viewpoint can help you deter-mine whether your high standards are healthy or destructive.

I have done my best and it is enough.

—AFFIRMATION FOR PERFECTIONISTS

STEP 2: LEARN TO RELAX
take a deep breath

When we are stressed and tensed, we breathe shallow, rapid breaths. Make a daily habit of tuning into your breath and taking slow, deep breaths throughout the day. Before dealing with a stressful situation, stop and take a few deep breaths. Deep breathing helps cleanse and supply the body and brain with life-giving oxygen. It will also help you regain clarity and focus for facing the challenge at hand.

In many cultures, the terms used to describe spirit and breath are the same. The breath is considered a bridge to spirit. The term *spirit*, derived from the Latin word *spiritus*, means "the breath of life." *Ruh* in Arabic and *chi*, also spelled *qi*, in Asian cultures are all similarly used to describe a vital yet invisible force of energy that flows within us. In yogic philosophy, *pranayama*—breathing exercises—are practiced to calm the mind and body, increase concentration and access and control (*yama*) the flow of vital energy (*prana*).

Yoga teacher Angela Cerkevich, CYT, states that in times of stress and anxiety, sometimes the most affective technique for calming the mind is not simply breathing deeply but actually retaining the breath. She suggests the following breathing exercise, called *Kumbhaka*, to restore natural, deep breathing and concentration (Please note, Kumbhaka should not be practiced if you have hypertension, heart disease, asthma and ulcer):

1. Sit comfortably, with an erect spine. Close your eyes.

2. Observe the rhythm and quality of your natural breath, without attempting to change it. Watch for where and how you feel your breathe in your body.

After three to five minutes of this, take a deep breath, inhaling for four counts.

3. Hold your breath for four counts. Then, fully release your breath, exhaling for six counts.

4. Repeat this breath retention four to eight more times. After this, take time to observe the quality of your breath and changes that may have occurred. For added calmness, imagine an image of peace while retaining the breath.

move your body

By their very nature, our bodies' natural fight or flight responses to stress require physical movement. Physical activity helps the body metabolize excess stress hormones in the bloodstream. Physical activity also stimulates the release of endorphins, feel-good biochemicals that give us a sense of general wellbeing. (A more detailed discussion of the benefits of physical activity is provided in principle 5.)

Walking, especially in nature, is the ideal prescription for stress. By stepping outside with an eye toward observing and appreciating the beauty of your surroundings, walking physically transports you away from your everyday demands. Walking can be a meditative exercise that brings clarity, calm and a greater sense of connectedness to God and yourself. By taking time to soak in the beauty of nature's sounds, fragrances, birds and other elements that animate our world, we appreciate the natural order and flow of things—a stark contrast from our culture of over-stimulation, resistance and determination to make things happen. Nature reminds us that there is a delicate balance that we must observe and strive to maintain between our inner and outer worlds.

call upon friends and family

We know instinctively that friends and family can be a source of comfort and relief in times of distress. As a result of new research on how women cope with stress, scientists have found that women have a special survival mechanism. In addition to "fight or flight," women often call on the natural urge to "tend or befriend" when under stress.

Oxytocin, a stress hormone released by the pituitary gland to calm the body during times of stress, makes women care for their children or seek out family and friends. It is the same hormone that is naturally secreted to aid in childbirth. While men also produce oxytocin, the effect isn't the same because testosterone reduces oxytocin's effectiveness. In contrast, estrogen enhances oxytocin's calming effect. We have all experienced this response at one time or another. When something stressful happens we seek out our best girlfriends. Teenage girls run to the bathroom to talk after an embarrassing incident at school. It's the built-in female advantage to stress.

While the news on "tend or befriend" is recent, the link between social support and mental health is well established. Our ties to friends and family can significantly enhance the length and quality of our lives. One study found that among women with symptoms of heart disease, those who had smaller social circles were twice as likely to die than those with larger social networks. In the study, social circles encompassed relationships with family, spouses, friends, coworkers and community groups. The quality, not just the quantity, of relationships mattered. This is an important point since some relationships may in fact drain our energy and add to our stress. Thus, the message is that we should seek out relationships that energize instead of drain us, that enhance our wellbeing instead of diminish it.

Good friends are there to hold our hands, cry with us, support us and enrich our lives. We should all have at least one person we can turn *to talk about* anything under the sun. When we can't physically see each other to connect and benefit from our friendships, a phone call can do wonders.

Nobody sees a flower, really, it is so small.
We haven't time – and to see takes time like to have
a friend takes time.

—GEORGIA O'KEEFFE

smell the roses

When was the last time you stopped to smell the roses? Essential oils have long been used for treating a variety of conditions including anxiety, insomnia, respiratory congestion, and, of course, stress. These oils, usually derived from flowers and plants, can also elevate mood and relax tense muscles by stimulating areas of the brain and nerve endings on the skin that elicit emotional responses. Readily available at spas, health food and department stores, essential oils can be used in a variety ways:

- **Inhaled.** Place a few drops in a diffuser or in a bowl of hot water. With a towel over your face, lean over the bowl and breathe. Essential oils also come in mists that you spray in the air and on your face, hair and body. One of my favorite mist scents is Gingermint from Aura Cacia. Mists usually have water in them, so they are not as potent as pure oils—

which can me mixed to create a customized blend of oils specific to your needs.

- *In a Warm Bath.* Fill your bathtub with warm water, put a few drops of the oil in the bath and lie back and relax in the healing waters.

- *Massage.* Place a few drops of oil in the palm of your hand. Rub your hands together to warm the oil and massage it into tired and tense muscles.

Common Essential Oils for Stress Relief

Bergamot	Elevates mood, calms mind
Chamomile	Aids in sleep, relieves tension
Citrus	Uplifts and energizes
Eucalyptus	Opens congested breathing passages
Lavender	Promotes relaxation, aids in sleep
Rosemary	Stimulates mind and body
Sandalwood	Eases anxiety, aids in centering and grounding
Spearmint	Alleviates mental fatigue, clears mind

Georgia O'Keeffe, famous for painting flowers in grand scale, painted large flowers to grab people's attention, especially that of busy New Yorkers. Otherwise, she said, they would not see the flowers' beauty. But, O'Keeffe believed New Yorkers would be more surprised by the fact that they were stopping to take time to look at the flowers she had painted.

Fortunately, O'Keeffe's appreciation of the gift of flowers was not lost on a group of researchers at Rutgers University. The researchers found that the presence of flowers can trigger happy emotions and heighten feelings of satisfaction.

Consider keeping fresh flowers around as a symbol of your commitment to your health and wellness. They can also be a reminder of the beauty and simplicity of just pausing for a few moments to consciously breathe and be fully present. Keep them on your desk or somewhere you'll appreciate them, like in your living room. Let these small, conscious steps remind you that you're moving closer to fully blossoming into the well woman you desire to be.

let the music play

Music has a profound effect on mood. When we're stuck in traffic, the right music can calm us and make the time go by. At a party or social event, music can set the background for a mellow, intimate evening or an upbeat, all-night soiree. We choose upbeat music when we're out for a walk or jog, or calm, meditative music when we want to relax.

Music has been used for centuries for healing, meditation, celebration, mourning, spiritual awakening and prayer. Just about every human emotion and experience can be captured in sound. "Music expresses that which cannot be said and on which it is impossible to be silent," said Victor Hugo, the famed French poet, playwright and author of *Les Misérables*. From the ancient Indian tradition of chanting to the drumming of African tribes to American gospel singing, music is a bridge to the spirit. In Chinese medicine, chi—the field of energy that flows through every human being—responds to sound vibrations. "Certain sound wave vibrations can heal organs on the cellular level," says Dr. May Loo, Clinical Assistant Professor at Stanford Medical Center and author of *East-West Healing: Integrating Chinese and Western Medicines for Optimal Health.*

Through entrainment or synchronization, sound and music can change our brainwaves and states of consciousness. Entrainment is a simple physics principle which states that two or more rhythmic processes or bodies will entrain or harmonize with each other. A classic example of this is the synching of the menstrual cycles of women who live or work together. Music's effect on brainwaves can trigger changes to bodily functions controlled by the autonomic nervous system, such as breathing and heart rate. Slow, meditative music can induce a relaxation response, including slower breathing and decreased heart rate, blood pressure and metabolism.

Music is used therapeutically in hospitals and non-clinical settings to treat depression, pain, attention deficit disorder, cancer, and a host of other mental and physical illnesses and disabilities. It is also used to promote wellness, reduce stress, improve communication and enhance memory.

Although the power of music to stimulate our minds, bodies and spirits has often been referred to as the Mozart effect, you don't have to be a Mozart or classical music fan to enjoy the benefits of music. Classical, New Age and folk music have the best benefits, but you should use music that you enjoy. There are also brainwave CDs, such as the ones created by Dr. Jeffrey Thompson of the Center for Neuroacoustic Research, that are specifically designed to facilitate mental and physiological changes and objectives, such as creativity, deep relaxation, healing and problem solving.

Alice Cash, Ph.D., has been helping people use music for healing and wellness for over twenty years. When using music for stress management, Dr. Cash notes the following:

1. It is most important to use your favorite categories of music. If you don't like Mozart or classical music, don't use it! (However, I do hope you'll at least try it!)

2. Choose music that has pleasant associations for you, music that brings you cheerful memories.

3. Because it does not require you to "think," instrumental music tends to be more stress-relieving than music with lyrics.

4. Racing thoughts can lead to anxious and stressed-out feelings. For this reason, use the rhythms of slow music to slow your body and thoughts down. Dr. Cash also recommends music that has a regular pulse or beat. Researchers have discovered that music with the tempo of the healthy, resting heartbeat will guide (synchronize or match) your own breathing and heartbeat to it, thus slowing down our racing body rhythms.

A Poem for Beauty and Balance

Silent Beauty

Silent beauty be still

Silent beauty be still
under the tree

Silent beauty be still
under the tree
focused on me

Silent beauty be still
under the tree
focused on me
and you will see

Silent beauty be still
under the tree
focused on me
and you will see—
arrows become beautiful flowers

principle three

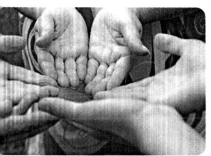 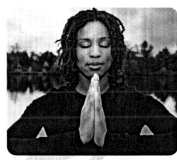 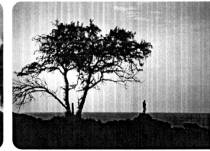

feed your spirit

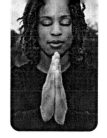

Spirit

Spirit is the heart of living well, the center of our health and wellbeing. It is an ever-flowing well and source of life, love, energy, health and beauty. Stripped down of all that defines us in this world—down to our very core—our spirit is the one thing that remains. Your spirit is your true nature, connected to a higher creative and intelligent power that unites us all. It is "home base" and the only true source of inner peace.

When nurtured, our spiritual lives bring us peace and grounding, even in the midst of life changes and challenges. Nurturing our spirits builds our inner strength and resources like intuition, creativity and tenacity—essential tools for modern living. When we feel connected to our Source, our lives always have meaning and purpose. When we feel disconnected we experience a deep sense of longing and dissatisfaction, as if something is missing or "just isn't right." To compensate for this lack, the ego, our lower self, tells us that we need more: more friends, more money, more recognition, greater achievement, more food and more clothes, jewelry and material possessions. But we can't fill our emptiness and longing for love and meaning by feeding ourselves with external substitutes. In contrast, when we are aligned with our highest selves, we are in tune with our true needs. We know what feeds us and we know what makes us whole.

Your spirit is your inner reservoir of wisdom, calling you to return to your self, the part of you not occupied with doing, but just being. The part that knows surrendering to a power higher than ourselves makes life easier and more fulfilling.

Individual happiness is the foundation for creating peace in the world.

—THICH NHAT HAN

make the connection and commitment

We are all on this journey to our higher selves both individually and collectively. Buddhist philosophy teaches that if we cultivate peace within ourselves, we cultivate peace in the world. When we nurture the light within, it shines without. We become more radiant, more beautiful, more patient and more loving. As we share our patience, gratitude and love with others, we send positive energy out into the world that can inspire hope and healing. By taking care of ourselves, we are taking care of the world. The world needs more happy and whole women shining our light and using our power to affect change, if even in the most subtle ways possible.

It may seem strange and even selfish to focus on ourselves with such devotion, but when we look at our health, happiness and personal development as a contribution to the world, it changes things—at least it did for me. I always considered myself to be an advocate, to be a woman who was concerned about others and the world. But the thought that my greatest contribution to the world could be my wholeness and freedom, well that takes it to another level. If I could live to my fullest potential, how would that change me and the people I touch? It is a call to live with greater integrity. To "be the change." To be better healers, we have to heal our own pain and wounds. To be compassionate caregivers, we have to show ourselves compassion, love and patience. Imagine how much better the world would be if we all took our spiritual development and wellness as seriously as we took going to school and being employed. We would have healthier families, safer communities, compassionate institutions and more socially responsible businesses.

When women lose touch with their real selves, the harmony of the world ceases to exist, and destruction sets in. It is therefore crucial that women everywhere make every effort to rediscover their fundamental nature, for only then can we save this world.

—MATA AMRITANANDAMAYI (AMMA)

Whatever your spiritual tradition or beliefs, we can agree that spirituality is the glue that holds us together. It enriches our lives and connection to each other, nature and the Divine. There are innumerable ways that we can nurture our spirit. Some of us touch Spirit through church attendance, service to others, creative expression or being out in nature. Anything that is done with conscious and loving intention can be a spiritual act. Eating and exercising mindfully. Reading inspirational books or journaling. Volunteering, playing with your kids or retreating to a hot bath. Whatever you believe and however you choose to develop your inner life, find a way to nourish this special part of you every day. Tending your spirit is good medicine.

live your values

One of the best ways to nurture your spirit is to live your values. Values are enduring and consistent. They are a core part of who we are. Living our values keeps us focused on the path to living our healthiest and fullest lives. When you know what you value, it's easier to make decisions that honor who you are, while saying no to people and situations that compromise your values. Using my core values as a guide helps ensure that I am doing the right thing for me. When I am in a situation or environment that doesn't honor my values, I look for the door because I know that is not where I want to be for long. I may be fine for the short-term, but I know that I will need to find a way out before long. I also use my values to decide what types of projects and contracts I accept and pursue. I don't work for companies or organizations that contradict my core value of health. And since I've reprioritized my time and values, I don't accept projects that will make it difficult to maintain my own health and peace of mind.

> 60
>
> The percentage of Americans who believe that spirituality is involved in every aspect of their lives.
>
> 70
>
> The percentage of Americans who state that their lives have meaning because of their faith.

Let the beauty of what you love be what you do.

—RUMI

We are always expressing our values. Everyday we make choices that hint at what we care about. Where we work, who we work with, what we eat, where we shop, how we spend our time—these are all opportunities for our values to be expressed and shared with others.

The list of values below will help you hone in on your values. Select the ones that really "speak" to you. This is not a comprehensive list. If there's a value that resonates with you but isn't on the list, feel free to add it. Once you've done that, narrow your personal list down to three to five values. Go a step further and prioritize them. A good way to drill down to your core values is to ask yourself, *What would I fight for? What do I absolutely need to have or experience to say that I have lived a good life?*

Spirituality is the center of my wellness. My connection to God has gotten me through loss, parenting, being a psychotherapist—all of which I could not have done alone.

—CONNIE, AGE 65

The priority that you place on certain values can shift over time. For instance, success might be on the top of your list in your twenties, but love may take precedence in your forties. Or you may have an experience, such as a major illness, that shifts your thinking and consequently your values.

love	nature	purpose
health	beauty	control
faith	opportunity	connection
security	power	equality
peace	freedom	intimacy
success	service	diversity
wealth	energy	passion
fame	happiness	creativity
family	truth	change
simplicity	respect	justice
education	compassion	kindness

Another way to identify your values is to revisit the "vision of wellness" exercise in the first chapter. What do your responses tell you about your values? Are you living them? If not, how will you start integrating them into your life? For example, if health is on your list, consider whether your food choices, level of physical activity and self-care practices are reflective of the value that you place on your health?

journey into silent bliss

The more we simplify our lives and build pockets of silence and tranquility into every day, the more we open ourselves to experience the wonders of the world. When we quiet the "noise"—including desires to stay busy, watch TV or seek fulfillment through other distractions—we invite the silent, still voice of Spirit back into our lives. It is always with us, inside and all around us.

Lying or sitting in silence can be peaceful and comforting once you get used it—and it can take some practice! By temporarily abandoning clocks, watches and alarms, we experience—in silence—the gentle flow of time and ourselves flowing along with it. With TVs, radios, and cell phones off, we can fully experience the beauty that surrounds us.

Silence allows us to reintegrate ourselves, helping us to feel whole again. Some of my most peaceful and life-affirming moments are enjoyed in silence, listening to the sounds around me. The sound of the ceiling fan circulating air in the room. The voices of people passing by or children playing outside in the distance. Birds chirping. Trees blowing in the wind. In silence, I appreciate the sun that shines brightly in my living room. I feel and appreciate the order of the universe. I know that God is with me.

Looking around the room, I can appreciate the beauty of pictures, furniture, pillows, candles and other objects. In an open and organized space, I am reminded and grateful of the purpose and functions of the objects around me. They hold, reflect, beautify, illuminate, comfort, support and tell stories.

sitting in silence to appreciate the beauty and blessings of life is a silent prayer and act of devotion.

In moments of silence, time doesn't slow down. Instead, we slow down for time. Time is open. It's graceful. Accepting. Anything can happen in a moment of time. Time waits to be filled with sound, light, action and life. Time is ever-present, always moving fluidly and silently.

When enough of us learn how to become deeply, profoundly quiet, then the hysteria of the world will begin to subside.

—MARIANNE WILLIAMSON

The serenity of silence is always available to each of us. Even the busiest among us can steal away for quiet time. Five minutes here, fifteen minutes there, can make all the difference in your life.

Are you ready to take your own journey into silence? Try these six steps to find your silent bliss:

1. Think of your quiet time as a way of centering yourself. It is also a way of saying grace. Sitting in silence to appreciate the beauty and blessings of life is a silent prayer and act of devotion.

2. Find a quiet and comfortable place to sit where you will not be disturbed

3. Take in a few deep breaths. Relax and let go.

4. Allow yourself to be completely present in the moment. Observe the sounds inside or outside your space but do not allow them to pull you from your center—where you are at the moment. Try not to think about what you have to do, what happened earlier in the day or anything unrelated to your present experience.

5. Look at the things around you with an eye of appreciation. Try to see the beauty of everything around you and the higher good and purpose they serve in your life. If you prefer, choose to focus on one object—its color, shape, texture and function in your life.

6. After a few minutes of this, close your eyes and observe how you are feeling. Open your eyes when you're ready to return to your daily activities.

BE MINDFUL

Be grateful. Give thanks for the blessings in your life. Choose to see the good and abundance in your life, being thankful for what you have right now.

Be present. Practice meditation, sitting in silence and other mind-body-spirit exercises, such as yoga. They will ground you in the present moment, enhancing your ability to appreciate the beauty in everyday occurrences and encounters.

Be kind. Start with being kind to yourself. Honor yourself by nurturing your spirit every day through prayer, meditation and other ways that connect you to the things and people you love. Cultivate love, peace and kindness within, then share it with the world.

go inward with meditation

The word "meditation" is derived from the Sanskrit word *medha*, which means "wisdom." For a long time I resisted meditation because I didn't think it was something I could do, but then I learned I could design my own meditation practice in a way that fit me. I encourage you to do the same.

Meditation is seen by some women as inaccessible and unappealing. Understandably, it may be hard to slow down and sit in silence when you are used to running around and multitasking. I recently suggested meditation to a friend who was wondering why she couldn't lose weight. She was under a lot of stress, so I suggested to her that she incorporate more deep relaxation methods to counter her body's stress response. When I asked her if she meditated, she sarcastically responded, "Yeah, I meditate!" But when I suggested finding pockets of tranquility throughout the day, even just five minutes to meditate, it seemed more reasonable. The longer the better, but even a few minutes can be helpful. I love the alternative that internationally renowned Buddhist monk and meditation guru Thich Nhat Hanh offers. According to Hanh, the ultimate goal of meditation is to teach us to be more mindful, that is, more present in every moment. He gives the wonderful example of how washing dishes, if practiced with complete mindfulness, can be a form of meditation. Meditation can also be practiced through movement during yoga, dancing and walking. Knitting, which is enjoyed by many women, is also a meditative practice. The repetitive movements of the hands in knitting a scarf or sweater can induce a state of deep calm and contemplation that women use to meditate or "knit prayers" for loved ones.

The key is to find what works for you. Yoga is the core of my meditative practice. I attend a class once a week and practice at home as part of my morning routine. After my yoga practice at home, I often do a heart meditation to open my heart (see principle 4). I also use a guided meditation CD weekly and dance to music that moves my soul. In yoga, the poses are largely practiced to prepare the body to stay still in meditation. By balancing the energy in the body, you are less like likely to feel the need to fidget or move around during meditation. In fact, after a good yoga session, all I want is to lie or sit still, basking in the serenity and sense of calm derived from my practice.

Meditation is taking you deeper and deeper inside yourself, until you reach the area untouched by illness. This is a very real part of yourself.

—DEEPAK CHOPRA

Traditional meditation involves concentration on an object, word, mantra or movement of breath while sitting in an upright position. As you develop your personal meditation practice, you will discover that there is value in both seated (or lying down, which I prefer) and moving meditations. All forms of meditative practices have one goal in common: to quiet the mind so that the truth of who we really are is revealed.

Meditation helps to calm the storm of our thoughts and emotions, giving way for us to fully experience the present. While meditating, instead of resisting or judging thoughts and emotions, you observe them. Observing our thoughts teaches us that *we are not our thoughts*. Focusing on an object, word or movement during meditation anchors the mind in the present. The more we experience "mindful moments" through meditation, the more present we become in other moments throughout the day. A regular meditation practice will bring you to a state of peace and harmony. It is from this place of harmony that we access inner guidance, mental clarity, creativity, vitality and new insights about ourselves and life's challenges.

Personally, meditation has made me more accepting and patient. I am less irritated by waiting in traffic or in line at the grocery store. Shortly after developing a regular meditation practice, a colleague saw me at the supermarket and noted how relaxed I looked. During several events that we'd worked on together, she would often say to me, "You look worried." or "You look stressed." At those events, I could never enjoy myself or be fully present because I agonized about how everything would turn out, what the attendees were thinking, or how things weren't going as planned. I no longer suffer through events in this way.

Physically, meditation calms the nervous system, eliciting a relaxation response that reduces blood pressure, heart rate, breathing rate and muscle tension. It can also boost the immune system, slow down aging and alleviate symptoms of depression, anxiety, premenstrual syndrome (PMS), menopause and a host of other health conditions.

You might be thinking, "Meditation sounds great, but I don't have the time to do it." You do. You don't need a lot of time to meditate. If you're just starting, begin with five minutes. If you would like more information on meditation, look for a class, workshop or teacher that teaches techniques in line with your spiritual beliefs. Books by the Dalai Lama and Thich Nhat Hanh offer great instruction on how to meditate for an open heart and other spiritual qualities, such as compassion and forgiveness. I also like *Meditation Secrets for Women* by Camille

Maurine and Lorin Roche. It's filled with light-hearted and unconventional recommendations on how to design your own meditation techniques. For now, you may want to try the Silent Bliss exercise described above or try the two simple meditations below:

- *Five-Minute Meditation.* Take five minutes, wherever you are, to notice your breath or simply pay attention to how you are feeling in your body. Place your hands on your abdomen and notice how it moves up with each inhalation and down with each exhalation. Don't try to change the rhythm of your breath, just notice it. Imagine your thoughts floating away like balloons. Be gentle and patient with yourself. Don't expect to stop all your thoughts at first. You might find yourself wondering about that meeting at 4:00 PM or what to cook for dinner. If your mind starts to wander, gently return your focus to your breath. As with all disciplines, meditation will get easier with practice. As you begin to experience the benefits, you will want to lengthen your sessions.

- *Enchanted Meditation.* If you're at home and have more time, take a few minutes to silently relax and prepare for your meditation, creating an experience that invites you to relax and go deep within. Try to meditate in the same space or location each time. Your sacred space should be quiet and, if possible, not used for any other purpose. Your mind will associate your sacred space with a state of peace the more you meditate there. Wear comfortable, loose-fitting clothes. Light a few candles. You may want to play soft music that draws you inward. Use a mat or cushion to sit or lie on. Rub a few drops of an essential oil in your hands. Inhale and/or massage into your temples, third eye (center of your forehead), neck and chest. If you like, say a prayer for peace or guidance. Sit with your feet crossed or lie down on your back, palms up. Sitting upright will keep you from falling asleep. If you choose to sit, place your hands on your lap or knees, palms up. Take a few deep breaths, and then focus on your breath, mantra or object of concentration. If your mind starts to wander, gently return to your focus. Be patient with yourself and trust that over time you will get better at staying focused. Don't expect any magical or transformative experiences, but be open to them if they do happen. Just be in the moment. Continue for five to twenty minutes. When you are ready to come out, slowly begin to wiggle your fingers and toes, fully bringing yourself back into your body. Open your eyes. Your session is complete.

walk in prayer/walking meditation

Walking is one of our most basic instincts. As toddlers, we instinctively stop crawling and start stumbling on our two feet until we finally reach one of the greatest achievements of our early life—to put one foot in front of the other and walk! For those of us that can walk, it's hardly the crowning achievement it was when we were toddlers. We forget that our feet ground and connect us to the earth. We even abuse our feet in the pursuit of beauty and style. As our foundation and as tools for propelling us forward, our feet are sacred instruments for navigating the world around us.

Walking is so natural and automatic that often, while walking, we arrive at a destination without any awareness of what happened during the journey. Our thoughts pull us away from the experience. But when we walk for spiritual nourishment, walking takes on a whole new meaning. We can walk for enlightenment and clarity. We walk to places of meaning and significance, such as a church, synagogue or our homes. We can walk a labyrinth for contemplation and insight or walk a garden to commune with nature. Walking takes us out of our cars and places us in the midst and mystery of the sky, earth and rivers. There is an energetic shift that happens within us when we walk. It shifts our attention and changes our perspective. Being outside—even in an urban environment—can remind us that we are part of a greater whole, something larger than ourselves. Nature can remind us that while we may not be able to make sense of it, there is an order to things. Sometimes that order is much like walking—it is successive, beckoning us to take one step at a time.

Whoever you are, no matter how lonely, the world offers itself to your imagination, calls to you like the wild geese, harsh and exciting—over and over announcing your place in the family of things.

—MARY OLIVER

Instead of thinking about your worries or the details of the day, transform your next walk by making it a meditative or prayerful experience. If you find sitting still in one place difficult, this form of meditation may be a good starting point for you:

1. Concentrate on your steps, such as how and when each step hits the ground. Start off walking much slower than your normal walking pace. This will force you to be conscious of the movements of your feet and hands.

2. Become aware of your breathing. Hanh recommends saying "in" to yourself with each inhalation and "out" with each exhalation.

3. If you find concentrating on your steps and your breath at the same time to be cumbersome, choose an affirmation, prayer or word—such as *love, peace or surrender*—that has a special meaning. Repeat the affirmation, prayer or word during the entire walk. If your mind wanders, bring your attention back to the powerful words that you have chosen to concentrate on during the walk. One of my favorite affirmations for walking is, "I know where I am going, and I know what I'm doing." This is an excellent affirmation for times of uncertainty or when you need clarity.

If you can't get outside, modify your walking meditation by walking the perimeter of the room or wherever there is space for you to walk without objects blocking your path.

find inner harmony through yoga

Dating back more than five thousand years, yoga is a holistic and practical system for living. It encompasses asanas (poses), meditation, philosophical and spiritual teachings, and Ayurveda, the ancient Indian healing science.

Practicing yoga unifies all aspects of the self. Through concentration, movement and breath, yoga brings you fully into your body. The poses and breathing exercises release tension, increase flexibility, improve balance and synch mind, body, heart and spirit. Because yoga stimulates glands, nerves and organs, the poses and breathing exercises also balance hormones and heal a host of physical ailments. Rodney Lee, one of the foremost experts on yoga, likens the various poses to airing out an attic. The movements help pump experiences like depression, grief and stress through the body, says Lee.

The difficulties and stress of everyday life are often absorbed in our bodies and manifested through bad posture, muscle tension, increased heart rate and high blood pressure—all of which can be improved through the regular practice of yoga. For the past twenty-five years, Dr. Dean Ornish has helped patients reverse advanced heart disease through yoga, meditation and a low cholesterol diet. Yoga is also effective in treating and alleviating the symptoms and effects of a number of health conditions including depression, arthritis and breast cancer.

Far more than just physical exercise, at its core yoga is a path toward self-discovery—a way to deeply know yourself. In yogic terms, to know yourself is to know God. A journey to freedom and personal power, yoga frees life energy and builds strength for everyday living. Through yoga poses we celebrate our greatness, allowing our spirits to shine through conscious and expressive movement. With each pose, yoga gently pushes us to open ourselves in new ways, to make space for grace and lead with our hearts. It teaches us to be patient, poised and present both in our practice and in life. It brings the seemingly disparate parts of our life together by focusing our mental, physical and spiritual energies. The focus, synchronicity and grace developed on the mat become guiding principles for aligning and living our lives from our core.

Yoga is a practical philosophy. It shows, from moment to moment, the way to face the world and at the same time to follow a spiritual path.

—BKS IYENGAR

To truly live well, we must be willing to bring all aspects of ourselves into alignment with our true nature. The guiding principle of Anusara yoga, the form of yoga that I currently practice, is that our highest intention is to "align with the Divine." I did not fully grasp this concept until I began practicing regularly at home. Yoga has always been useful in helping me address my chronic muscle aches, but since committing to a regular yoga practice, it has become an incredible resource for balancing my emotions and nurturing my spirit. I have gone to yoga class and cried on the mat because of the emotional release I experienced during my practice. It has provided more than an ideal—it gives me a foundation for living.

As I embarked on my own transformative path, doing the inner work of healing emotional wounds, realigning my life and priorities, and letting go of the things that I thought defined me like success in my business and work, yoga grounded me as parts of myself disintegrated. As I made yoga part of my morning routine, it was no longer just about feeling better physically but about touching a core part of me that had been neglected. Each time I brought my hands to my heart while doing sun salutations, I was filled with a sense of gratitude and devotion. My practice became a prayer. A prayer for wholeness. A prayer for freedom. A prayer to live and rest in God's love.

Traditionally in the United States, the spiritual aspects of yoga are down-played to make it more acceptable. But there is something in yoga for everyone. I have found, like many others, that yoga has strengthened my faith—and it will strengthen yours, regardless of what religious or spiritual tradition you are rooted in. Yoga is not a religion, but its teachings are parallel to the great religions of the world, like practicing *ahisma* (non-violence), *satyam* (truthfulness), *brahmacharya* (moderation in all things) and *asteya* (non-stealing).

There are many forms of yoga. Some emphasize physical fitness while others focus on precision of poses or spiritual development. You will need to find the one that best meets your mental, physical and spiritual needs. The more common forms include: *ashtanga* or "power yoga," gentle yoga, Iyengar yoga and Anusara yoga. Anusara yoga teaches that we are each perfect expressions of the divine, regardless of how we express a certain pose.

I also enjoy the Yoga Trance Dance and moving meditations of Shiva Rea on DVD. Hers is one of the few pre-set DVD sessions that I really get into at home. Shiva's style is more of a flowing dance designed to "liberate your creative life force." It's an energizing way to meditate and express your spirit through dance and movement.

If you haven't tried yoga, the best way to learn is by attending a class. Books, DVDs and videos are great supplements but can't take the place of live instruction. Classes also have the added benefit of forcing you to leave your everyday environment, which may be stressful, for an opportunity to retreat and commune with others who share your values.

surrender in prayer

Prayer reconnects us to the source of our energy and life. Prayer reminds us that we are not alone—that we are not separate from the power that created this universe. When we pray, we acknowledge that we don't have to take on the burdens of the world and the challenges in life by ourselves. We acknowledge that as wise as we may think we are, there is still a wisdom much greater than our own.

In prayer, we surrender to the will and power of divine love. In our keep-fighting–and-pushing world, surrender is often considered a sign of weakness. But surrender is an act of faith and strength that positions us to see things with new eyes. It centers and opens us up to receive and appreciate our blessings. Prayer,

> *I take time daily to appreciate the unlimited abundance in my life. I realize everything is in Divine Order, regardless of how much I think I'm in charge.*
> —BRENNA, AGE 57

as the saying goes, makes a way. When we are in a constant state of resistance, we work far harder than we need to. Resistance tightens and closes. Surrender opens and invites.

Melissa West, a psychotherapist and spiritual counselor to cancer patients, says that surrender is not giving up, but giving control of our lives back to God. "For the past five years, I have witnessed participants in Harmony Hill's cancer retreats surrender to the mystery of their journeys and offer a passionate and unreserved Yes to life even in great pain and uncertainty," says West.

Prayer is one of the most common alternative health practices, according to a study conducted by the National Institutes of Health National Center on Complementary and Alternative Medicine. Sixty-two percent of American adults pray specifically for health reasons. Prayer is a universal source of healing, comfort, joy and guidance. We pray for ourselves, for loved ones and strangers. We pray for health and healing, for understanding and for change. We sometimes wonder whether our prayers are answered. We may not get what we ask for, but the answer to our prayers can come in mysterious ways. In Neale Donald Walsch's book *Conversations with God*, we are reminded that the answer to our prayers can come in the next song we hear, article we read or movie we watch. It may even come "in the whisper of the next river, the next ocean, the next breeze that caresses your ear."

With a growing interest in the connection between spirituality and health, there are many studies looking at the effectiveness of prayer as a healing modality. But we are wise not to wait for a study to validate our prayers. Besides, can we really predict God's actions? And how can we measure the effectiveness of a limitless power? These are questions being debated by the scientific and spiritual communities. Many of us know the power of prayer to change and heal in even the direst circumstances, and in challenging times, our lives may rest on a hope and prayer. Still, there have been several clinical trials showing the positive benefits of distant prayer on health. What is interesting about the studies on prayer is the effect it has on the person praying. The studies by Harvard cardiologist Dr. Herbert Benson have shown that meditation and prayer trigger a relaxation response: slower heart rate, lower blood pressure, slower breathing and lower metabolic rate. The key is repetition of a mantra or prayer like "Hail Mary, full of grace" for Catholics or "Shalom" for Jews. Benson has also found that people who are spiritual—not necessarily religious—are more likely to be in better psychological health and have fewer stress-related symptoms.

We can create our own rituals around prayer, such as praying in the morning and at night, while in the shower, before a meal or while exercising. Our prayers don't have to be complicated or structured. They just have to come from the heart. A prayer can be as simple as a heartfelt "thank you." We can also find comfort and inspiration in the poetic prayers of spiritual leaders we respect, and may keep them near during times when our spirits need uplifting. We can pray at any time of the day or when we are moved by spirit, joy, pain or grief in ourselves or in others. In any form, our prayers are creative sparks that reconnect us with divine energy. We are free to completely be ourselves in prayer.

Give yourself freedom to pray with a creative spirit. Speak, sing, dance, paint, knit or write your prayers.

principle four

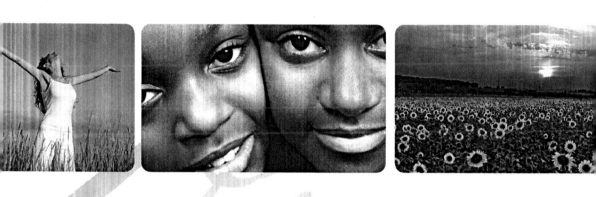

open your heart

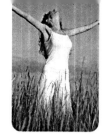

The heart is the eternal and sacred space within us that reflects both our humanity and spirituality. The heart is where all four levels of our being—mind, body, spirit and, of course, heart—meet. We have an emotional heart that needs to experience love, joy and passion. There is also the built-in intelligence of the heart that serves as an inner compass or guide (you might call this intuition). Physically, the heart pumps vital blood throughout the body. Spiritually, the heart is universally recognized by as having a direct connection to Spirit and other people. We "give from the heart" and love "from the bottom" of our hearts. When we cultivate qualities like kindness and compassion for ourselves and others, we learn to speak the heart's language. That language is love: love of self, others and life.

Research by the Institute of Heart Math is now providing scientific evidence of what most of us know instinctively: the heart is a sensory organ with its own brain. It is comprised of 40,000 neurons, just as many as the brain in our heads. The heart continuously sends signals to the brain that affect our perceptions, thinking and emotional processing. The heart's magnetic component, according to the Institute, is about 5,000 times stronger than the brain's magnetic field and can be detected several feet away from the body. Like the brain, the heart can entrain to other electromagnetic fields and rhythms, such as the hearts of a couple or of a mother and child beating in unison.

The loving heart is our share of the true, good, and beautiful—something genuine to cherish and venerate.

—LAMA SURYA DAS

When we are living from the heart, we're radiant. It's how we know that our girlfriend has fallen in love. The glow from her heart is like a ray of sunshine. This is not a fairy tale, head-in-the-clouds notion either. Cardiology research tells us that the rhythm of our heart beats changes in response to our emotions. When we are frightened, our hearts beat faster. When we are relaxed, they beat slower. According to The Institute of Heart Math, the heart's rhythm is smooth and ordered when we experience positive emotions. Our bodies work more efficiently and we experience greater emotional balance. In contrast, when we experience negative emotions, the heart's rhythm is erratic and less coherent. The longer we remain in a harmonious, positive state, the more we tap into our innate vitality, creativity, intuition, sensitivity and connection to others.

closed hearts and blocked emotions

The Upanishads, an ancient Sanskrit scriptural text, compared the "little space" within the heart to the vastness of the universe. The text goes on to liken the heart to other parts of nature, "The heavens and the earth are there, and the sun and the moon and the stars. Fire and lightening and winds are there, and all that is and all that is not."

The heart has the capacity to hold an immeasurable amount of joy, pain, guilt, passion and other emotions. It is like a bowl or a cup that never fills to capacity, never runs over—unless we decide to close it. We may close our hearts when we have been hurt by loss, grief, betrayal and disappointment. But even when we close our hearts, they desire to be reopened. The heart's natural state is to remain open so that we can continue to give and receive love. Love sustains us. The blood that flows in and out of our hearts is a symbol of that love. It nourishes every part of our being.

But when we're hurt, we may decide to not venture down love's or hope's path again. We all go through this at some point. Something happens that so devastates or disappoints us that we resolve to never do it again or never come close to anything that resembles or reminds us of that situation or person. We are wounded and hurt and close our hearts and minds to anything that would cause us to relive the painful emotions and experiences. In that closing, we can become filled with anger, bitterness and resentment.

Emotions are energy in motion. When that energy is bound up or buried inside, it blocks our ability to see and experience the innate health, beauty and joy in and around us. Our senses are dull. We feel disconnected from people and the world. With closed hearts we are unable to trust, love, give, care or see the good in other people. We hold on to past hurts, unable to release them and move forward with our lives—they color everything, and we are unable to experience things as they actually are.

When we are out of touch with our emotions, life isn't as it should be because, regardless of how hard we may try to deny it, it is human nature to be emotional beings with emotional needs. Bestselling author Gary Zukav notes that, "The longest journey that you will make in your life is from your head to your heart." Many of us live in our heads, using worrying and busy-ness to avoid our emotions. But the path to wellness has to go through the heart.

My tears don't compromise my strength.

—KATRINA SURVIVOR

As women, we are often in conflict with our natural tendency to be emotional, believing that it's a sign of weakness or vulnerability. We are also told that we should experience only one emotion—happiness. Women aren't supposed to be unhappy or sad, so we "put on the happy face" when our hearts are really breaking. Repressing our emotions won't make them go away. They are real and they stay with us, in one form or another. Prolonged exposure to or repression of emotions like fear and anger creates disharmony in the mind and body that can later show up as chronic aches and disease. In contrast, positive emotions experienced over time, as previously mentioned, result in increased vitality, health and inner harmony.

When we suppress our difficult emotions, we are interrupting the natural flow of energy in our body. The muscles in the neck, shoulders, back and chest are often places where suppressed emotions get buried or lodged. Emotions often come to the surface during massage and other types of bodywork. Therefore, bodywork and body awareness are essential parts of emotional healing and growth. When we are conscious of how our body responds to emotions, we gain insight on how we process our emotional experiences. Tension and tightness may suggest that we are stuck in holding patterns and have difficulty letting go or expressing ourselves. These patterns are often learned early in life, for instance, when well-meaning parents or caregivers tell children to "stop crying." Over time, when we find that we don't have a safe outlet or environment for expressing our emotions, suppressing them becomes a *normal* response. But we know this is not a normal or healthy approach.

Babies have a lot to teach us about expressing our emotions. Under normal circumstances, babies cry uninhibitedly. A crying baby will cry with her whole body, expressing her emotions or discomfort through sound, breath, physical movement and tears.

If one is out of touch with oneself, then one cannot touch others.

—ANNE MORROW LINDBERGH

build your emotional health toolkit

We have become so skillful at hiding our feelings, even from ourselves. In my own experience, I have suffered for several years with chronic muscle tension. I have tried all kinds of mind-body therapies for resolution. But in my search, I have developed an awareness of my body and emotions that has been an unexpected gift from my physical discomfort. When I feel emotional tension and blocks in my body, I release them through deep breathing, massage, yoga and journaling. Sometimes just placing my hand on the tense area for a few minutes brings a heightened sense of awareness to my emotional needs at that moment. Although I had considered psychotherapy previously, it was in one of the those moments just described that I finally decided to move forward and actually seek therapy.

One evening, I felt a heavy feeling in the center of my chest. I had been working all day in front of the computer. Nothing about the day seemed to trigger any obvious intense feelings in me, but as I wrapped up my work for the day I could not ignore the physical sensation that I felt near my heart. I knew it was an emotion, but I couldn't name it. So I sat on the floor in my bedroom, concentrating my attention on the tightness. I began to moan. I had learned from an energy medicine practitioner to release emotions through sound. Sound is an incredibly useful tool for accessing and expressing emotions. At times, naming what we're feeling may be hard, but if we can express this feeling through moaning, singing, chanting, humming or whatever is appropriate, the energy in the body shifts and creates an opening that allows emotions to flow through instead of getting stuck. As I moaned, I could feel the tightness give way to tears. It was not until after crying for several minutes that I finally understood why. I felt alone. Those old feelings of being alone and unsupported were bubbling up, and I needed help to finally begin to effectively move through them.

> *As for emotional stress, I walk if off, sing it off, cry it off, and then pray it off.*
>
> —ALFREDA, AGE 57

If you feel emotionally stuck in the past, consider seeking help. With effective tools and support for understanding and expressing our emotions, we can restore and maintain the healthy emotional balance that is so critical to our health and wellbeing. The next few pages provide tools and suggestions for building your own emotional health toolkit.

Learn to recognize your emotions. Do you know what you're feeling when you're feeling it? Your body will probably tell you far quicker than your mind. A good way to develop emotional awareness is to start taking note of how you feel physically when you experience both pleasurable and painful emotions. Does your heart beat faster or slower? How is your breathing? Do you feel tension or tightness in any part of your body? Underneath tension could be emotional pain, fear, frustration and anger. If you're anxious you might start sweating and your heart might beat faster, or your muscles may become tense. Sadness might be expressed through crying or feelings of fatigue. On the other hand, you might catch yourself smiling or feel an incredible sense of relaxation when you're happy.

If you are unsure of how you feel, try physically checking in with yourself. It's simple. Find a quiet place and lie down if there is a bed or couch nearby. Close your eyes and bring your attention to your breath. Don't try to change your breath, just pay attention to it. Now ask yourself, What am I feeling? Observe how your body responds to the question. Is there a part of you that seems to feel a heightened sensation? Or maybe it feels numb or dull? Bring your attention to that area and ask yourself again, *What am I feeling?* Can you identify or vocalize what you are feeling? It doesn't have to be words. It may be a moan or a sigh. Once you've identified the emotion, decide what you will do next. It may simply be to sit with the feeling for a while, observing and processing it. If you find yourself worrying or sinking into a state of despair, try some of the positive outlook strategies mentioned in principle 1.

Develop awareness of your needs. Emotions can be powerful energies or waves that move us to action. Far too many of us go straight to action, without allowing ourselves time to process the message that our emotions are communicating to us. When we take action without thinking, it is often destructive, such as yelling at, manipulating and hurting others in order to communicate our needs.

Our emotions stem from four primary needs that we all deeply want met:

- **Love:** To experience love, connection with and support from others

- **Respect:** To be respected, acknowledged and listened to

- **Freedom:** To share and express ourselves freely

- **Purpose:** To feel that our lives have meaning, purpose, and are in service to others

There are innumerable ways to have our need for love, respect, freedom and purpose met in life-affirming and constructive ways. Each of us has to figure out how to have these needs met in a way that honors ourselves and the people and world around us. A good place to start is by defining for yourself what these four needs would ideally look like in your life. They can also be applied to a variety of relationships. For instance, in a romantic relationship you might outline the following needs:

- **Love:** A mutually caring and affectionate partnership

- **Respect:** Where we honor each others' thoughts, feelings and needs and listen with an open heart and mind

- **Freedom:** I feel free to express who I am and pursue my dreams

- **Purpose:** To grow spiritually as a person and as a couple while nurturing and honoring each other's minds, bodies, hearts and spirits

After you have outlined your needs, think about the various ways you would like them fulfilled. What action will you take? What action will your partner, friend or family member need to take? Is it realistic in that they can meet these needs in the way you would like? If not, can you accept that they may not be able to meet your needs in the ways you desire? How do you think you might react if they can't? Sometimes we place the burden of our happiness on one or two people or one "big" idea. Do you need to lift the burden that you placed on someone and reclaim responsibility for your happiness?

Here are more questions to help you on your journey to emotional awareness and health:

1. Are your primary emotional needs being met?

2. What, if anything, do you say or do when you experience intense emotions like anger and frustration? Do these reactions support healthy emotional flow and balance? Are they constructive or destructive?

3. Have you closed a part of your heart off?

4. What happened to cause you to close your heart?

5. How has closing off your heart (or other parts of yourself) affected your life?

6. Are you missing out on something or someone because your heart is closed?

7. How can you open your heart and allow all of God's blessings to flow freely in your life?

8. How can you begin or further your emotional healing?

9. Do you need to reach out for help?

Develop healthy emotional responses. As part of the natural flow of movement through our bodies, emotions have to be experienced and processed in healthy ways through the many forms of expression available to us. It is important that we arm ourselves with a toolkit for dealing with emotional and stressful events. Along with other emotional skills, your toolkit might include expression of your feelings through:

- **Voice:** speaking, journaling, singing, chanting, moaning, humming, etc.

- **Physical Activity:** dancing, yoga, and other forms of physical activity

- **Breathing:** breath awareness, diaphragmatic and other deep breathing exercises to calm and relax the body

- **Meditation:** seated, walking, and other forms of meditation

- **Psychotherapy:** talking to a licensed professional such as a psychologist, social worker or counselor. Therapists with a mind-body-spirit orientation may use massage, deep breathing, physical exercises and body awareness to help you access your emotions.

- **Bodywork:** a variety of methods for working with the body's energy fields, muscles and tissues including various forms of massage, Rolfing, Reiki and healing touch

As you assess what combination of tools you will use for your emotional health, think about how you currently respond to emotionally stressful events. Your responses will be mostly determined by your personality and temperament. Some people are highly sensitive while others may be largely unaffected by the same emotional or environmental stimuli. According to Elaine Aron, Ph.D., author of *The Highly Sensitive Person*, 15 to 20 percent of the population has highly sensitive personalities. Highly sensitive people (HSP) are more easily stressed out, overwhelmed and overstimulated. As a result, HSPs need to withdraw in stressful situations and even arrange their lives to avoid upsetting situations. For HSPs, crowds, loud music and even electromagnetic waves from computers and other electronic devices can be unnerving. This sensitivity, says Aron, is not a weakness; once understood it can be used as a strength for dealing with a variety of life challenges. In the book, Aron provides useful suggestions for protecting your energy and taking better care of yourself when alone and with others.

Whatever your personality, physically withdrawing from a stressful situation can be the best way to keep your cool. Remaining in the situation or environment keeps your body in fight or flight mode and can cloud your judgment. In this case, taking a walk and/or a deep breath can be the best thing to do. Physical activity can assuage anger and give you a new perspective on the whole situation.

When you get angry, stop and ask yourself what need isn't being met. Do you feel that you're not being listened to? Respected? If you find an argument or conversation becoming stressful, ask for time to gather your thoughts and resume the conversation when both of you have had time to think. Alternatively, if you become angered by something someone said or did, it may not be appropriate, or you may not be ready, to speak to the person that angered or hurt you. But don't hold on to anger. Anger is a destructive emotion and can wreak havoc on your health when not appropriately channeled.

Learning how to express our needs, wants and disappointments is necessary for healthy self-expression. If you determine that you can't tell the person how you feel, find another healthy outlet for dealing with your emotions. In this instance, activities like yoga, meditation and journaling can be a great help. Speaking to a trusted friend is always good too. But don't keep replaying the stressful event—doing this can actually stimulate a stress response—exactly the opposite of what you want.

Several years ago I remained in a stressful job for far too long. While searching for a new job, I stayed at my current one despite being passed up for a promotion which I, along with everyone else, thought I would have been a virtual shoe-in for especially since I was already doing the work required of the new position. But what upset me was the underhanded manner in which the director of the department went about denying me an interview. I was angry and told everyone but her. Because she violated the organizations internal hiring rules, Human Resources and the Executive Director of the organization became involved in the whole affair. Long story short, I stayed in the job six months after the incident and at times had to travel and conduct three-day workshops side by side with her. All of this while neither of us said one word about the entire incident! A few months before I finally left, I had the most painful episode of muscle spasms that I have ever experienced. A day after attending a two-day department retreat with the director and other staff, the spasms started and I could barely move my right arm. I made the connection immediately. The whole time during the retreat I was internally fuming over her repudiated commitment to justice, fairness and equality. If she was so committed to these values, I wondered why she would treat me and other employees in the way that she did. Regardless of her apparent contradictions, the issue was with me. I was still upset about what had happened six months earlier and was suffering for it.

Whether positive or negative, emotions are transformative. We can use them to move further or closer to our higher selves. As such, we do ourselves a great service when we unload the emotional baggage that weighs heavy on our minds, heart, body and spirit. We also give ourselves the gift of harmonious living when are conscious of our emotional needs. When we are aware of our emotional needs, we are empowered with the knowledge of what makes us feel more alive and what makes our hearts sing.

Your emotions are messages designed to help you find the love, respect, freedom and purpose you need. Starting today, give yourself permission to listen. By acknowledging, accepting, and, when appropriate, taking constructive and loving action to have your needs met, you'll move closer to the life you were meant to live.

Watch over your heart with all diligence, for from it flows the springs of life.

—PROVERBS

six ways to open your heart

An open heart is a healthy heart. When we open our hearts, we experience positive emotions that create balance in our lives. Our hearts beat with coherence and harmony. The brain receives and processes these positive messages from the heart and synchs our thoughts, emotions and actions—giving us a greater sense of clarity, peace and wellness.

There are so many ways to keep your heart open. Here are just a few of them:

1. Forgive and let go. Holding on to past hurts is detrimental to our health. The various emotions that block forgiveness, including anger, hostility, resentment and fear, can lead to stress, which is further linked to obesity, increased blood pressure, disruptive hormonal changes, impaired immune function and heart disease.

It can seem nearly impossible to forgive a wrong, but we can find solace and inspiration from individuals who have reminded us that the human heart has the capacity to forgive even the most atrocious and inhumane acts. Consider Immaculee Illigabiza, who hid for sixty days in a bathroom to escape torture and certain death at the hands of Hutu rebels during the Rwandan genocide. Immaculee says that during those days she prayed for her life and found God. While she wanted to hate those who would have surely killed her had they found her, she found it in her heart to forgive them. To hear her speak about the terror and her personal triumph over hatred is a moving testimony to the spirit of forgiveness.

> I keep my heart open by surrounding myself with youth. They haven't been tainted by the disillusionment we often face as adults. Plus they keep me on my toes!
>
> —STARR, AGE 25

Stories like Immaculee's may make your pain seem small. It isn't. Emotional pain can imprison us in ways that make release and forgiveness seem impossible. Yet if we are willing to work through the process of forgiveness, it is possible. Robert Enright, Ph.D., author of *Forgiveness is a Choice*, describes forgiveness as a "matter of a willed change of heart, the successful result of an active endeavor." That means that we have to work at it. Most of us can't simply forgive just because we say or decide that we want to. Yet setting the intention is an important first step toward releasing guilt and shame that you may be harboring toward yourself or others.

Only through accessing the power of the Now, which is your own power, can there be true forgiveness. This renders the past powerless. . .nothing you ever did or that was ever done to you could touch even in the slightest the radiant essence of who you are.

—ECKHART TOLLE

To benefit from forgiveness, experts suggest adopting a personality of forgiveness rather than seeing it as something we do in response to a particular incident. You can begin to develop a forgiving personality by learning to let go of everyday gaffes (such as a friend showing up late or a stranger maneuvering into a parking spot at the mall despite the fact that you were there first). If you make a mistake, accept it as such instead of beating yourself up about it. If you have been deeply hurt by someone else's actions, take time to process the experience and your emotions. Be patient and compassionate with yourself. Allow yourself the time that you need to heal. Seek the help of a mental health or spiritual counselor if you need assistance with the forgiveness process. Forgiveness is not easy. Pray for guidance and the gift of forgiveness. *To err is human, but to forgive, divine.*

Here are a few questions to consider in your journal if you are working toward forgiving someone:

- Have you faced your anger or pain? How has the event or injury affected your life?

- How is holding on to resentment, guilt or blame serving you?

- Did the "offender" intentionally mean to hurt you?

- Does he/she know that you have been hurt?

- Do you want to forgive the person?

- Do you want to reconcile or be reunited with the person? Is reconciliation an option? Would it cause more suffering?

- Can you pray or wish for the best for the offender?

- How can you turn the wound into wisdom?

2. Inspire Your Heart. I am often awed and inspired by people like Mother Teresa, who seemed to have an unending capacity to love. Closer to home, my grandmother's ability to love and care wholeheartedly, not just for family members but also for others in need, is an inspiration. An immigrant from Haiti with an entrepreneurial spirit, she paved the way for my parents to migrate to the United States. Though she has seven kids of her own, many people, myself included, have also been mothered and cared for by my grandmother. She is a role model, showing me how to love, to open my heart and keep it open, even though life may be tough or filled with disappointment and pain.

During times when we struggle to keep our hearts open, we can find inspiration from spiritual teachers, leaders and people in our lives who were able to tap into their heart's immense reservoir of love and compassion to passionately serve and help others.

Just watching other people do good acts can have a profound, heart-opening effect. Recall the example mentioned in the first chapter where students were shown clips of Mother Teresa. An open heart can inspire and touch many in ways we can't imagine. In much the same way, our lives can inspire others.

3. Be of service. We can serve, love and give back to others in infinite ways. When we help others, it reminds us of our own humanity and interdependence on each other. Service also fills us with a sense of purpose and a means to make a difference.

There are countless examples of women who transformed emotions like grief, anger and frustration into positive action. They have taken the message from their emotions to start organizations, to volunteer and raise awareness about a myriad of issues including domestic violence, drunk driving, homelessness, AIDS, discrimination and more. If you're thinking, "I don't have time to give back on that level," trust that whatever way you find to give back is best for you. The key is to serve in a way that speaks to your heart. It is often the little things that have big impact. Help a friend or family member, serve food at a homeless shelter, help out at a food bank, or give a homeless person a few dollars to get something to eat.

Consider giving regularly to a charity of your choice. Regularly scheduled giving is a reminder to keep the channels of love and service flowing to and from your heart. Organizations like Save the Children offer the opportunity to sponsor a child in the United States or around the world for less than $30 a month. The donation helps not only the child but also his/her family. You also have an opportunity to develop a relationship with the child by sending letters and photos. If you've ever wondered who your charity dollars are actually helping, then sponsoring a child, woman or family through organizations, such as Save the Children, links you with the people you help. The companion Resource Guide for this book lists several respectable charitable organizations that you may want to consider supporting. The Guide is available online at www.heartandstylewoman.com

4. Be grateful. A popular French proverb reminds us that *gratitude is the heart's memory.* When we genuinely appreciate the many blessings and gifts in our lives, the feeling resonates in our hearts as joy. Age-old spiritual wisdom has taught that a grateful heart is key to happiness and health. Several studies have shown that people who adopt an attitude of gratitude—that is, they regularly appreciate the good things in life—are happier and more resilient. In one study, people who counted their blessings weekly for ten weeks noticed that they had fewer physical complaints, spent more time exercising and experienced improved quality of sleep.

These studies reinforce the benefit of shifting our focus to the good and positive things in life. Gratitude is a choice to focus on the good instead of the negative in our lives. It is also a choice to be present in the here and now, instead of in the past or future. When we are truly grateful, we are satisfied with where we are in the present moment. Unfortunately, in a high-pressure, results-driven society that tells us we should *want it all* and *want more,* being satisfied is mistakenly perceived as settling for less. But we can have goals and look forward to a future of bigger and better things while savoring and celebrating the blessings of today.

Gratitude is a higher level of consciousness. It is above the fray, so no matter what our circumstances, when we express and experience gratitude, the positive energy from feeling grateful reverberates within and around us. The law of attraction teaches that like attracts like. What we praise and appreciate grows, so if we are thankful for what we have, there will be more for us to be thankful for.

Life is a wonderful gift: family and friends, lessons and challenges, the wonder of the extraordinary and the familiarity of the everyday, the abundance and convenience of food we enjoy, our health, homes, jobs and businesses, the light of the sun, the magnificence of nature. There is already so much for us to be thankful for.

How do you express your gratitude? Here are few ways to build your gratitude practice:

- Say a prayer of thanks each morning

- Keep a gratitude journal

- Light a candle

- Pause and bring your hands to your heart

- Reflect on three good things that happened at the end of each day

- Send a thank you note

As travelers on a wellness journey, praising and expressing gratitude for our minds, bodies, hearts and spirits is essential. Embracing and accepting all parts of who we are right now opens the door for health and healing on all levels of our being. As part of your gratitude practice, regularly thank your body. Start at your toes and work your way up to your head. Thank your muscles and tendons for helping you move, your bones for supporting you, your blood for carrying oxygen and nutrients to your cells and tissues, and your heart, lungs and other organs for their respective functions.

5. Meditate on an open heart. Some of my favorite yoga poses are those specifically designed to open one's heart. Many of them are aptly called "restoratives." They gently relax the muscles in the upper back and around the heart, physically opening the heart. When we adopt a posture of openness, our hearts, minds and breath respond accordingly. Similarly, when our bodies are tense we become rigid and inflexible in our thinking and our breath is shallow.

Try this heart opener:

- Firmly roll one to two blankets (the blankets should be rolled firmly and evenly throughout).

- Position the blanket on the floor so that when you lie down on your back, it will run horizontally underneath your shoulder blades.

- Sit with your knees bent, and then lie down slowly on your back. Stretch your legs out. Adjust the blanket so that it is properly positioned underneath your shoulder blades. If needed, place a thin blanket or pillow under your neck for support.

- Stretch your arms out to either side of you with palms up.

- Relax and settle into the position for a few minutes. Bring your awareness to the center of your chest. Observe how it feels. Any tension you feel will begin to dissolve as you relax. Remain in the pose for a few minutes, focusing your attention on the center of your chest area.

- As you settle in, you can stop at the previous step or pray or repeat a mantra or affirmation for an open heart. It can be as simple as "love is flowing to me and through me," or a few lines from the "Open Heart" poem below. Or just observe your breath.

- Stay in the pose as long as you wish.

A Poem and Affirmation for an Open Heart:

Open Heart

My heart is open
wide open
open to life
open to health
open to peace
open to wealth

My heart is open
open to give
open to receive
open to live
open to believe

My heart is open
open to love
open to conceive
open to inspire
open to forgive
open to desire

My heart is open
wide open

6. Find your passion. Our passions excite and motivate us. Passion gives our relationships, work and life meaning. Our passions energize and continually refuel us. Fueled by love, passion is a feeling that comes from our hearts. When we live passionately, we live with the natural flow of our hearts. When we are in tune with our heart's passions, we allow our creative spirit to express itself freely.

Unfortunately, with our many duties and responsibilities, we often miss out on opportunities to engage our passions. We say we'll get to our favorite hobby one day "when there's more time," but there never seems to be. Recently, I met a woman who loves to paint but can't seem to make time for it. She acknowledged that she was retiring soon but that she still may not paint, even though she would have more time to do it.

Are you pushing your passions aside, hoping that one day you'll "have more time?" Our passions are so important to our wellbeing. We owe it to ourselves to enjoy them today. Our passions take us out of our heads and into our hearts. They enrich us and make us feel alive.

Don't ask yourself what the world needs. Ask yourself what makes you come alive and then go do that. Because what the world needs is people who have come alive.

—HOWARD THURMAN

What are you passionate about? What makes you excited? What did you love to do as a child? What have you dreamed about doing? What would you do if money were no object? These are useful questions to ask yourself if you haven't found your passion. Now is the time to find it. Give yourself permission to play, dabble and experiment. Step outside yourself and try something new. Maybe something that you never thought *you* would do. It might just be the thing that lights your fire.

journaling: a tool for your heart and spirit

A journal is a place where we can tune in to our mental, emotional, physical and spiritual needs. Journaling calls upon our inner wisdom and reveals our heart's desires. Writing in a journal allows us to focus on our deepest feelings, not just on events but also how these events, people and life experiences affect us. Journaling is a creative process, freeing us to express our thoughts and emotions through words, drawings, pictures, lists and more. When we pour our hearts and minds out in our journals, in many ways they become symbols of our lives, reflecting our thoughts, emotions, desires, dreams, pains and joys.

Keeping a journal will change your life in ways that you'd never imagine.

—OPRAH WINFREY

Journal writing is a great way to process and reflect on our lives. With the speed at which many of us live, years can go by before we realize that we are no longer living our dreams or that our dreams have changed. We can get caught up with fulfilling roles, performing routines and completing tasks, never taking time to consider our feelings or needs. During a teleseminar for our lifestyle coaching program, I was touched my one of the participants, who relunctantly shared with the group, "I am forty years old and I don't know myself. I have spent the past eighteen years trying to be a good wife and mother." Sadly, her feelings are far too common. As women, we often give of ourselves until we can't give anymore. We run out of fuel, passion and energy to care for ourselves. Yet journal writing is a simple self-care and self-discovery tool that can center and ground us amidst the changing winds and tides of our lives. Going back and reviewing old journal entries can provide insight on the changes and growth you have experienced, remind you of your passions and provide perspective on your life today.

Journals also reveal patterns of behavior, such as choosing men who are emotionally unavailable or emotional eating when you are stressed. Perhaps you've been telling yourself for months or years to leave your job or take a vacation. Looking back and seeing these patterns and the associated emotions can be a strong impetus for change and action. When we explore our lives through writing, asking ourselves essential questions of "who, what, when, where, why, and how," we open ourselves to the wonderful gifts of self-reflection, discovery and empowerment.

the healing power of journaling

The power of journal writing is real. Scientific studies show writing about emotional and traumatic life events can help us heal, strengthen immune function and improve chronic disease outcomes.

James Pennebaker, M.D., a researcher and professor at the University of Texas at Austin, turned to journal writing when faced with the stress of marital problems. He credits journal writing with allowing him to see his relationship with his wife in a new light, saving his marriage. After experiencing the benefits of journal writing, he decided to scientifically test whether journaling had an effect on health. Through his studies with rape victims and others who experienced traumatic events, he found that the immune systems improved among people who wrote about emotionally stressful events for just twenty minutes a day, for three or four days.

Choose how you'll write. The beauty of journaling is that it is a highly personalized, affordable and accessible activity. There are many options for journal writing, including journaling software programs you can install on your computer. One popular software program, LifeJournal, includes features that allow users to create a timeline of their lives, track health or energy levels, hours slept or miles walked. It also features a search function that pulls up diary entries by topic, date and journal type. Additionally, some women's websites offer users the opportunity to keep private journals.

The jury is still out as to whether you can achieve the same benefits from electronic journaling as traditional pen and paper method. When Palm Pilots first came out, I bought one, fascinated with the cool new device that would allow me to stay organized and be on the cutting edge. While I loved the phone book and quick note feature, I seemed to lose something in keeping my appointments and to-do list stored in the PDA. Writing them out would often store these details in my memory, and seeing them laid out in a physical calendar would allow me to access the information I needed more quickly. So as much as I am "up" on new technology, there are some things that I prefer the old-fashioned way, such as my Day Minder calendar and traditional hard-bound journal.

blog your life

Web logs, or blogs, are in many ways journals, albeit public ones. Blogs can be anonymous and offer a way to share your thoughts and emotions with others. For some, blogs can be therapeutic, allowing the writer to express herself with strangers in a way she might not feel comfortable with people she know. While reviving my own blog, I came across a blog started by a woman who wanted to vent about a guy who had been ignoring her calls. She was clearly upset with his behavior and felt that writing through the blog would help her cope. I've found that my blog is also therapeutic in a way. It allows me to comment on current events, giving me an outlet for expressing my voice and opinions on matters of public significance. With the limited access to mainstream media, many people, including women, are starting blogs as a form of self-expression and public commentary. Most of us have both a need for private expression of our thoughts and emotions through journals while also communicating them to others, be it face-to-face with friends and family, through cyberspace or by publishing articles and books.

Ready, set, write! An important first step in your journal writing journey is simply to commit to writing. You may not write every day; however, experts suggest that if you want to work through a major emotional event or trauma, you should write about that experience for fifteen to thirty minutes on three or four consecutive days. If you are suffering from major depression or a serious illness, you may want to speak with your therapist or doctor before delving into journaling. Writing about intense emotional experiences can trigger a stress response in the body.

If you are ready to start on the path of journal writing, here are few tips to guide you along the way:

- Decide how you'll write. Will you use a bounded journal, a three-ring binder or a computer? You may want to create separate sections for major areas of your life such as family, work, health, friends and goals.

- If you can't write or type, consider using a tape recorder or voice recognition software that allows users to dictate their thoughts to word processing and other computer programs.

- Write from your heart. Don't worry about grammar or spelling. Your journal should be for your eyes only, so you can pour your heart out, being honest about your emotions, thoughts and desires.

- Schedule a regular time for writing. Many journalers write before bedtime or first thing in the morning when they wake.

- Don't just record events. You will receive the most benefit by making a conscious effort to explore issues, events and relationships that have impacted or are currently impacting your life.

- If you are at a loss as to what to write about, start off by exploring your passions. Make a list of the things you love or the things you'd like to do in the near future. How can you begin to do these things? What has stopped you in the past? What's holding you back now and how can you move past the barriers?

- Be creative. Feel free to make your journal whatever you want it to be. Draw pictures of yourself or other people. Use colored pencils, markers or paper. Let your imagination run wild.

principle five

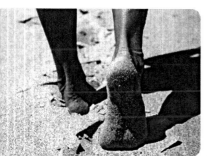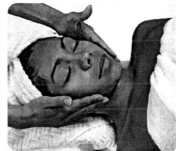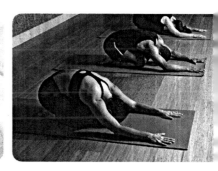

honor your body

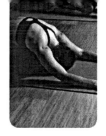

In nature, there is a constant movement of light, temperature, water and air that brings new life, renewal and change. The earth orbits the sun in just over 365 days. The sun rises in the morning and sets in the evening. As I write, snow is falling outside my window and the trees are barren. Yet, in a few weeks, the landscape will change as winter makes way for spring and new growth, just as it did last year and will again next year. Like the ebb and flow of the tides or leaves falling in autumn and returning beautifully in the spring, there is a continual give and take relationship that is also at work in our physical bodies. There is an innate wisdom flowing through us, guiding and directing us on how to best care for ourselves. Like nature, we are balanced through cycles and rhythms. The body's natural inclination is toward health. So when given the chance, it will work with nature's same trademark efficiency.

As rhythmic beings, we live in a constant flow of energy in and around us. The body itself is a complex energy system that is constantly seeking and maintaining equilibrium through regular bodily functions and processes. At any given moment, a rhythmic concert is being played within our bodies to sustain balance and health. On a basic level, we experience these rhythms in our need to play or move, rest, eat and sleep every day.

Our bodies hint at the miraculous creativity and intelligence that lives inside each of us. Our red blood cells completely replenish themselves every twenty-eight days. Our liver cells do the same every six months. At birth, we already have millions of eggs awaiting ovulation and the potential for fertilization. Our hormones "rise and fall" through menstruation, pregnancy and menopause, reminding us of the natural and cyclical processes that underlie our lives.

Let us first be as simple and well as Nature ourselves.

—HENRY DAVID THOREAU

As the home for our spirits, our bodies deserve to be treated with the highest regard. Unfortunately, our modern way of life has thrown most women out of balance and put us at odds with our bodies. Instead of honoring and respecting the body we're given, we push it to conform to a myriad of expectations and demands that are both personal and cultural.

We are given only one body to carry us through the journey of life, yet often we abuse, neglect and judge our bodies in the most inhumane ways. Many women treat their bodies like cars—not caring *how* they work, but that they simply work. We ignore it when it tells us that it needs sleep, rest, water and attention. We force it to keep going with caffeine, sugar, drugs and other substances. And when we have pain or get sick, we turn it over to doctors and other professionals who we think should know better or more about the body that accompanies us every minute of our lives.

The only expert on your body is you. Yes, medical professionals have highly specialized knowledge of the body that can be invaluable when we are ill or gravely hurt. But we too should have intimate knowledge of our bodies. Yet, many of us know very little about our own bodies. Knowledge of our bodies is not reserved for the highly educated and specially trained. We don't all have to go out and get medical degrees, but if we are serious about good health, we owe it to ourselves to get to know our bodies.

Culturally, we have found a strange comfort in judging and admiring other women's bodies and appearances. We absorb the definitions of what beautiful and healthy looks like and try desperately to fit a mold. At the same time, we reinforce love-hate relationships with our own bodies that start at a frighteningly early age for most girls in this country. The mixed messages about our bodies come from every angle possible: parents, peers, teachers, religion, strangers and media. *You're fat. Too skinny, dark, pale, short, tall. You're showing too much skin, not enough skin, your breasts are too small, butt too big.* And on and on. In our attempt to fit the current standard of beauty, we force our bodies through diets, starvation, surgery and countless other shortcuts and quick fixes. Mass media and one-size-fits-all solutions are not only impractical; they fail to honor the uniqueness of our bodies. When we fight against the basic nature of our bodies, we create imbalances that set the stage for illness, discontent and an endless cycle of looking outside of ourselves for achieving true health.

Uniquely designed to house our spirits, our bodies carry within them lessons on love, growth, faith and life.

Self-love is a fundamental requirement for good health. If we can't truly and deeply love, honor and respect our bodies and the wisdom within, how can we ever truly be well? Starting today, make a contract with yourself to honor your unique nature by listening to and trusting the wisdom that lies within. Agree to treat your body with unconditional love and gratitude. Treat it with the respect it deserves and give it what it needs most—loving care and attention.

love your body

Your body is a faithful and reliable companion, a friend that deserves the royal treatment. It is with you through thick and thin (in some cases, literally). The body that you have is the only one you'll receive, so learn to accept, nourish and love it just the way it is. That doesn't mean that we stop trying to strengthen or improve it, but that we approach our health and wellness efforts from a position of strength and reverence, rather than a position of fear, disdain, disgust or out-right hate. This might be a stretch for many of us, since we often make healthier choices from a risk- or fear-based model, choosing to make lifestyle changes only when we realize there is a real chance that we might get sick. Fear can be a pow-erful motivator, but love is even stronger.

Some of us may harbor resentment toward our bodies. Illness or chronic health conditions can make us feel that our bodies have betrayed us, but they haven't. These feelings are usually borne out of feeling "stuck" in a body that has made life miserable. In my own experience, I have felt frustration about the chronic tension and aches in my body. One day during an intense period of my "self-improvement plan," I sunk into a deep state of despair, believing that dying would be best because I would be free from the body that had caused me such anguish. But I had no intentions of dying; it just felt like I was. What I really wanted was to feel free. As I cried uncontrollably, I realized I was purging and releasing years of emo-tional pain and baggage. I have come to appreciate that there are important lessons to be learned through my body. Discomfort or pain can be signals of not just physical imbalances but also spiritual, mental and emotional ones as well. Learning to listen to the tension in my body has helped me become aware of the healing that needs to take place within me. It has also taught me the importance of building a spiritual foundation from which to live my life. Underneath all the tension was a deep longing and need to be loved and supported. Ultimately, the deep love and support we all seek is divine love. When we reconnect with this love, the journey we make through our lives and through our bodies will be much easier.

I found God in myself and I loved her ...
I loved her fiercely.

—NTOZAKE SHANGE

Right now, begin to cultivate a spirit of gratitude and love for your body and begin to make peace with it. Develop a new vision for your physical self. Appreciate the connection that you have to the loving power that animates the world. Let go of the suggestions that anyone else might have made that your body wasn't good enough or beautiful enough. Our bodies were wonderfully and beautifully made to carry out a far higher calling than to meet the standards and expectations of others.

Can you appreciate and love your body for the way that it is today? For how it has carried you through the many phases of your life? For the lessons that it has taught you? Is your body trying to teach you something right now, like self-acceptance? Self-expression? Self-love? Can you love it, even if there is a hard lesson for you to learn through illness or chronic pain? We can't always control what happens to our bodies. There are environmental and other causes that have an impact on our health. But by building a positive belief system based on love, we give ourselves a fighting chance to recover or improve our health when faced with illness. Your body is a powerful instrument of communication that thrives when you live in loving relationship with it.

Four Ways to Start Loving Your Body Today

There are so many ways to love your body. Here a few to get you started:

1. Commit to giving your body the best care it needs, when it needs it, including ample rest, food, water, massage and physical activity.

2. Make a habit of thanking your body at night for supporting you through the day.

3. Journal or create a list of the ways your body serves you.

4. Lovingly touch and massage every part of your body from head to toe. Linger in the parts that ache and offer words of love and healing, such as, "Even though you are aching (or tight or hurting), I completely love and accept you." Do the same for areas you have disliked. For most women it's usually their breasts, butt, hips or thighs. Try, "Even though I have not always thought of you with love, I completely love and accept you."

5. Bless your body with loving intentions, affirmations and thoughts. Affirm that love, health, beauty and harmony reside in every one of your cells, in your blood, bones, muscles and organs. Envision love as a light moving from the top of your head down through every part of you.

tune into your body's wisdom

One of the simplest ways to tune in to your body's wisdom is by being fully present in your body. This is also one of the best ways to tune into your emotional and spiritual needs. The awareness you gain from fully being in your body will inform your eating choices and self-care efforts in profound ways. You'll begin to make more conscious choices that deeply nourish and satisfy your entire being. For instance, instead of eating something because it looks good or because it's something you always eat, you'll begin to intuitively recognize whether it's something that your body needs at that particular moment. Don't be surprised if you find yourself naturally avoiding sweet and fattening foods or anything that makes you feel heavy in your body. You'll start naturally gravitating toward certain foods, exercises and practices. When you can really feel yourself inside your body, you become powerfully attuned to the needs of your spirit—and you will hear it speaking as you make healthy lifestyle choices with a surprisingly effortless ease. I'm not saying you will completely overhaul your diet and life overnight. But the awareness you gain will create a subtle shift in your behavior that will pay big dividends in the future. I have personally noticed this shift in myself the more time I spend consciously listening to my body, with nothing to cover up what I am feeling such as caffeine, sugar or even a heavy meal.

> *I've learned, and am still learning, to listen to those little "red flags" that let me know something isn't right.*
> —SYLVIA, AGE 54

To tune into your body's wisdom, try this exercise:

Lie on your back on a comfortable surface like a bed or yoga mat. Place your arms to your side, palms up. Start at your left toes. Observe how they are feeling. Then move to the ankle, lower leg and thighs, pausing each time to notice the sensations both on the front and back side of your body. Observe how the whole left leg feels. Is it aching, tight, loose? Ask yourself why it feels this way. Be open to what answers pop up, such as, "I am feeling stuck." Move to the right leg and do the same thing, starting at your toes. Now bring your attention to both legs. Just feel both of them, together. Move up to your pelvic area, to your abdomen, chest, arms, palms and fingers. Keep pausing as you move through each section of your body. Move your attention up to your throat and up to your face and head. Once you've moved through all the sections of your body, feel your whole body together, as one form. Continue to do this for as long as you feel necessary. Just lie there, feeling completely present in your whole body.

caring for your body through diet, movement and rest

The previous section was designed to help you look at your core beliefs about your body. Hopefully it helped you look at your body in a way that supports and honors your spirit and your life. How we feel about our bodies is directly connected to how we care for ourselves. Our beliefs lay the groundwork for making choices that support our commitment to good health. If we are to experience the health and wellness we seek, a belief system grounded in love and respect for our bodies is a must.

If you're reading this book, it's safe to assume that you care about your health. It's also probably safe to assume that you are already doing *something* to optimize your health. My personal experience and work in public health have taught me that most of us know what we need to do stay healthy. Most of us know that at the very least we need to eat well, get enough rest, and stay physically active. These three basic steps are essential for a healthy lifestyle. All three speak to the natural rhythms that support us daily. They are not luxuries. They're necessities. We know that when we don't do these things, we suffer. We feel sluggish and heavy. We're unable to think clearly. We lack the vitality and energy to perform at our best. All areas of our life can be affected simply by what we eat, how much rest we get and whether or not we move our bodies enough. Through the neurotic pace of our daily lives, we have somehow turned these simple pleasures into dreaded inconveniences. Of course, nothing could be further from the truth. So let's stop the excuses. Now is the time to begin to experience the joy of a well-cared-for body. It all starts with simple choices made day by day to create a lifetime of good health. If you're just getting started with living a healthy lifestyle, know that it is never too late to begin taking better care of your body.

eat wisely

Food has a special place in our lives. It is a symbol of blessings and bounty. Food has a unique way of bringing people together; even strangers with seemingly nothing else in common can find unity in enjoying good food with one another. Whether we eat alone or in the company of others, food is a gift that nourishes our entire being. A properly balanced diet fuels us with energy and vital nutrients that sustain and enhance our health.

We all have an intuitive sense of when and how much we need to eat. When we tune into this inner wisdom, we eat in ways that benefit our health and increase longevity. In contrast, when we eat mindlessly or out of tune with our body's wisdom, we tend to overeat and make food choices that can damage our health. Our digestive systems also become 30 percent to 40 percent less effective when we mentally tune out while eating. Unconscious eating can ultimately diminish our vitality and lead to excess weight gain or chronic diseases like diabetes and heart disease.

So why are we eating mindlessly when we have an internal guide directing us on how to best eat? There are many reasons, especially social and environmental cues, that cause us to disengage from our inner wisdom. Below, you'll find tools and tips for addressing the main causes of mindless eating by relying more on your intuition to make wise eating choices. While I am not one for blanket dietary recommendations, there are some universal eating principles we can all benefit from. When practiced, you'll find that these recommendations will make eating more enjoyable and natural while enhancing your health and longevity.

1. Eat mindfully. Mindful eating simply means eating with greater awareness. When we eat with awareness of what we are feeling, we are less inclined to overeat or eat emotionally. By applying the principle of mindfulness to eating, we can develop a healthier relationship with food and in turn make healthier choices.

To maximize time, we often eat while doing other tasks. We eat on the go, at our desks at work, while driving or when watching TV. But when we eat mindfully, eating becomes the main event.

If you have never sat in silence and enjoyed a meal free of distraction, now is the time to try it. You'll be surprised at how much more enjoyable and nourishing a meal can be when you simply focus on eating and not on reading, talking or engaging in another activity. Approach your entire eating experience as a form of meditation. Set an intention or say a prayer to shift your focus to the food in front of you. Look at the food. What do you notice about the colors? What about the aroma? Eating is a sensory experience. Soak it all in. Put some food in your mouth and then put your fork or spoon down. What do you notice about the texture and temperature of the food in your mouth? Chew slowly, breaking every piece of food down into the smallest bite possible before swallowing and placing more food into your mouth. Savor every minute and every morsel!

As enjoyable as the above exercise is, the point isn't for you to eat this way all the time. Practicing this eating meditation a few times a week will help you become more aware of what you're doing and feeling while eating. You will also slow down when eating, which has major benefits. It takes approximately twenty minutes for your brain to get the message from your stomach that you're full. Eating slowly allows enough time for your brain to get the signal before you eat more than you need. By slowing down your eating pace you are less likely to overeat and more likely to feel satisfied when done. Thoroughly chewing your food will also make digestion and absorption of nutrients much easier.

2. Listen to your body. Healthy infants are naturally attuned to their hunger cues. They eat when they are hungry and stop when satisfied. As they grow, they learn to stop listening to this internal wisdom. Studies show that children's ability to self-regulate their food intake will diminish as parents try to control what their kids eat. Along with this early conditioning, dieting, skipping meals and regularly pushing off eating due to stress or lack of time has caused many women to stop listening to their hunger cues. When we ignore hunger signals, the chance that we'll overeat increases as we move from feelings of hunger to starvation. Skipping meals also sets our internal survival mechanism into high gear. When we skip meals, our metabolism slows down, and instead of using fat, the body stores it—exactly the opposite of what you want to happen if you're trying to lose weight.

Sustenance is one of our most basic physiological needs. Because feelings of hunger tell us when and how much we need to eat, learning to listen to our hunger cues is an important part of eating wisely. Trust your instinct to determine when you are hungry. Tell-tale signs are hunger pangs, rumbling in your stomach, loss of energy, a slight headache, trouble concentrating and irritability. If you are not sure that you're hungry, drink a glass of water. Thirst can often mimic hunger. Or try rating your hunger on a scale from one to seven where one is "starving" and seven is "full or stuffed." The goal is to eat when you are moderately hungry (two and a half) and stop when you're moderately full (five and a half). You might find it simpler to tune into your intuition by taking a few calming breaths and asking yourself a few questions, such as, *Am I hungry? What do I want? What would satisfy me?* You can also reconnect to your natural hunger cues by keeping a food diary. Keep track of the times you feel hungry. Note whether your feelings were triggered by time (Do you usually eat at certain times during the day?), environment (As soon as you get home?), social situations (When you're with your friend Karen?) or emotional triggers (When you feel stressed or bored?)

3. *Be portion savvy.* We are so blessed with an abundance of food in the United States that many of us take advantage of—consciously and unconsciously. We eat not only because we're hungry, but because we can. In the age of super-sized meals and extreme portion sizes, most of us eat more than necessary to stay healthy. Compounding the larger portion sizes is the belief that we should eat everything on our plate. Somewhere in our development, a well-meaning parent or adult probably told us we should eat all our food because there are starving kids in Africa. But we can't help hungry kids by eating more than our bodies need.

The mere presence of a bigger portion size may cause you to overeat regardless of how good the food may be. In a Cornell University study, moviegoers were offered stale popcorn in medium- and large-sized buckets. Moviegoers who were given the large buckets ate 34 percent more popcorn, even though they said it didn't taste good. When it comes to eating, our eyes are often bigger than our stomachs. So when at all possible, put only what you think will satisfy your hunger on your plate. If you feel satisfied before eating all the food on your plate, save the rest for later. If you're at a restaurant, ask to have the remainder boxed. Don't let anyone (including yourself) pressure you into eating more than you need to. Familiarize yourself with food labels and serving sizes. You don't have to know the precise number of ounces that make up a serving size, but it's a good idea to have a sense of what a normal serving size looks like. For instance:

- 1 serving of meat, poultry or fish = a deck of cards or the palm of your hand (don't count your fingers)

- 1 cup of cereal = a fist

- 1/2 cup of cooked rice, pasta, or potato = a cupped hand or half a baseball

- 1 baked potato = a fist

- 1/2 cup of fresh fruit = half a baseball

- 1 serving of vegetables or fruit = a fist

- 1 teaspoon of peanut butter = the tip of a thumb

If you are used to eating big portions, these serving sizes might seem small. In fact, you might be surprised to learn that you are eating two to three times the standard serving size. But don't be discouraged. Compare how you feel after eating the larger and smaller portions. Are you still hungry after twenty minutes when you eat smaller portions? Do you feel more energetic after the smaller meal? Lethargic after the bigger meal?

4. End emotional eating. Because food has a way of soothing and comforting us emotionally, many women use it to cover up feelings of depression, stress, fatigue, boredom and loneliness. Used in such a way, eating becomes a distraction or a way to numb the pain in our lives. We also eat when we are happy or want to celebrate, so whether we are up or down, food has become a tool for coping with emotions, at least in the short-term. It temporarily eases and comforts but can't take the place of the spiritual or emotional nourishment we all need. Part of tuning in to our inner wisdom means recognizing when we are truly hungry. Listen to your body and recognize your emotional triggers. Are you really hungry when you reach for the candy bar, brownie or bag of chips? More often than not, you will crave comfort foods like the ones I just mentioned rather than an actual meal when you are trying to feed an emotional or spiritual void. If you are really hungry, have a healthy and satisfying meal instead of snacking. If you feel the urge to eat in times of distress or boredom, try going for a walk or calling a friend. Seek ways to address the pain you may be trying to avoid. Your emotions and cravings are sending you a message. Spend time trying to understand what that message means for your life. Is it time for a change? Do you need more balance? An outlet of expression? Do you need to learn to be with yourself? Is there a part of you crying for love and attention?

There are several options outlined throughout this book for physically, emotionally and spiritually nurturing yourself including meditation, yoga, journaling and reaching out to friends, family or a mental health professional. Try new ways to nourish and express yourself without using food. Take a bath, dance or paint. Begin to incorporate a few of these alternative coping mechanisms into your life. Make them a part of your emotional health toolkit. Instead of using food to distract you from your feelings, use these tools to help you deal with your emotions in healthier ways. Used regularly, they will help create a sense of wholeness and balance in mind, body, heart and spirit, giving you a firmer foundation for navigating the ups and downs in life.

5. Forget dieting. Women often lose connection with their bodies' intuition because of dieting. Diet plans and the important cautionary messages about the dangers of obesity have women running scared when it comes to food. For millions of women trying to lose excess weight, eating has become wrought with anxiety and guilt instead of bringing pleasure and satisfaction. Instead of trusting their ability to make sound health choices, many women live in fear of each meal. But we can't live in fear and be well at the same time. Dieting keeps us in a perpetual state of relying on someone else's guidance instead of our own. It also creates feelings of deprivation that can lead dieters to binge on "taboo foods." In contrast, once we eliminate the notion that certain foods are taboo or forbidden, we often lose interest in them.

Our goal should be a healthy lifestyle that includes eating a balanced diet free of guilt, shame and deprivation. The starting point for letting go of the diet mentality is self-acceptance and self-love. If you are working toward building a healthier relationship with yourself, be gentle with yourself as you embrace your true beauty and power. Your ego will put up a fight and want to preserve things just as they are. But your higher self, your true self, desperately wants you to step into the light of who you are. When we relax and stop battling ourselves, life gets easier and our choices become clearer—including how to best live our lives for health and longevity. If you harbor negative thoughts and emotions about yourself, confront them. Know that you are not ugly, disgusting or any other labels that you or anyone else may have ascribed to you. Remind yourself that you are a beautiful spirit in a beautiful body. Recognize that your body has a way of knowing, a wisdom of what's best for your own body, including how much you will weigh. Respect and honor the totality of who you are. Lovingly care and feed your body, mind, heart and spirit. In time, you will notice a dramatic difference in the way you look and feel if you regularly engage yourself in the wellness practices outlined in this book.

6. Eat fresh, seasonal and organic foods. Nature is the best guide for healthy eating. When we eat foods closest to their natural state, we get the best nature has to offer in terms of nutrients, energy and flavor. Food that is locally grown and in season takes less time to get to the supermarket, creating less of a need for preservatives or processing. Because they are more readily available, seasonal foods are more economical too.

Eating in harmony with the seasons is a natural and instinctive way to eat. Our bodies are sensitive to changes in seasons and our nutritional needs change, thus seasonal foods are more in tune with our body's cyclic needs. Additionally, by eating seasonally we introduce a wider range of nutrients and foods into our diets—two benefits that are essential for good health. Personally, there's something special about enjoying pumpkin, sweet potatoes and all the warm spices like ginger and nutmeg in autumn or enjoying a light salad and occasional ice cream cone in the summer. The seasons often serve as the backdrop for elaborate celebrations that feature seasonal foods, such as thanksgiving dinner in November and the smorgasbord at regional festivals honoring every food imaginable, including okra in South Carolina, crab in Maryland and dates in California.

Seasonal foods will vary in different regions of the country, but here are some basic guidelines for optimal nutrition:

Spring: Look for tender, leafy green vegetables, such as spinach, romaine lettuce, and Swiss chard and herbs like parsley and basil.

Summer: Choose light, cool foods, such as strawberries, pears, apples and plums and vegetables, such as broccoli, summer squash, cauliflower and corn. Peppermint and cilantro are great summertime herbs.

Fall: Lean toward harvest foods such as sweet potatoes, carrots, onions and garlic. Choose more warming spices, including ginger, peppercorns and mustard seeds.

Winter: Look for root vegetables, including carrots, potatoes, onions and garlic along with corn and nuts.

As you shop for fresh seasonal foods, consider buying organic. Organic foods are produced without harmful chemicals that can cause damage to our bodies and environment. Organic foods are becoming more readily available,

> *Food, Glorious Food*
>
> *Eating is a natural part of life. Most of us in the United States are fortunate to be able to eat every day. That is not the case for many people around the world. As we become conscious of the things that we need to stay healthy, our awareness calls us to eat consciously, being mindful that food is a divine gift from nature and the countless people who grow, transport, prepare and cook our food.*

even in conventional supermarkets, as demand grows for fresh and chemical-free food. Organic food is sometimes more expensive, so if you can't afford to buy all organic, weigh your options.

The Environmental Working Group, a non-profit research organization, has developed a list of the most contaminated fruits and vegetables. The list was comprised using data from over 40,000 tests for pesticides on produce by the U.S. Department of Agriculture and the U.S. Food and Drug Administration. Consider buying organic when shopping for the twelve most contaminated items on the list, which have a particularly high level of pesticide residue: peaches, apples, nectarines, strawberries, cherries, pears, imported grapes, sweet bell peppers, celery, spinach, lettuce and potatoes.

We've been eating pretty much all organic foods–produce, eggs, grains, meats–for the past thirty years. At sixty-one, I am in perfect (glowing) health and feel wonderful every day– just as I did at thirty!

—JO-ANN, AGE 62

It's also a good idea to consider organic dairy products, such as milk, cheese and yogurt and organic meats and poultry. Organic poultry, dairy and beef products come from chickens and cows that have grazed on pastures that have not been sprayed with synthetic chemical pesticides or given antibiotics and hormones. There is also emerging scientific research that suggests organic milk contains more Omega 3 fats, vitamin A and vitamin E than non-organic milk.

make food your medicine

Hippocrates, the ancient Greek physician, once aptly declared, "Let food be your medicine." Today, with the major causes of death—including heart disease, diabetes and cancer—being linked to poor nutrition, there is tremendous value in making food our primary source of preventive medicine. While we each have individual nutritional needs, the following guidelines will help you choose foods that preserve and promote optimum health.

1. Determine your unique needs. Your nutritional needs will vary depending on your age, weight, lifestyle, health status and health goals. Your needs are unique, so you should have a customized nutrition plan designed just for you. A nutritionist can help you determine which foods will be best. Consider which foods give you energy and which foods sap it. Are there foods your body does not process well or outright rejects (such as dairy or wheat)? Do you need to change your diet to manage an existing health condition? Use the answers to these questions and your inner wisdom to help you and your nutritionist develop a plan for you. As you search for a nutrition advisor or plan, you may want to consider Ayurveda, the ancient Indian approach to mind-body health. In Ayurveda, every individual is treated differently according to his or her *dosha*, or basic constitution. The system is based on the idea that what each of us needs to survive is determined by our basic nature, which informs choices about which diet, exercises and medical interventions are best for us. In Ayurveda, diet is the foundation for health, healing and balance. Depending on your constitution, some foods create imbalances while others can maintain or help to restore balance. Contact an Ayurvedic physician or specialist for a private consultation.

2. Eat at least five to nine servings of vegetables and fruits each day. Fruits and vegetables are low in calories and provide essential nutrients and fiber. Five, let alone nine, servings may sound like a lot, but one serving is smaller than you might think. Examples of a serving include one cup of leafy vegetables, six ounces of 100 percent fruit or vegetable juice or half of a banana. Eating fruits and vegetables can provide a protective effect against heart disease and stroke, control blood pressure and cholesterol, prevent certain types of cancer, improve digestive health and prevent age-related conditions, such as cataracts and macular degeneration. Fruits and vegetables are the best source of phytochemicals, powerful micronutrients that may slow the aging process, boost immunity and lower the risk of heart disease, cancer, stroke, high blood pressure, cataracts, osteoporosis, and urinary tract infections. Choose a wide variety of fruits and vegetables including dark green, yellow, orange, blue and red sources.

3. Choose whole grains. Choose whole grain rice, bread, pasta and cereal instead of processed or refined carbohydrates like white rice and sweetened cereals. Refined carbohydrates, such as white rice, pasta and bread as well as white potatoes and high-sugar foods, can cause spikes in blood sugar that can lead to weight gain, diabetes, heart disease, and other chronic disorders. In contrast, at least three servings a day of whole grains may reduce the risk of diabetes and heart disease and help you maintain a healthy weight. In a recent Swedish study, women who ate more than four and a half daily servings of whole grains were one-third less apt to develop colon cancer than those who ate less than one and a half servings a day. Whole grains are high in fiber and are rich sources of B vitamins, such as thiamin, riboflavin, niacin, and folic acid. B vitamins help the body release energy from protein, fat, and carbohydrates and are essential for a healthy nervous system. Whole grains also contain antioxidants and vital minerals, including magnesium and selenium. Magnesium is used in building bones and releasing energy from muscles while selenium protects cells from oxidation and is important for a healthy immune system. Read labels to make sure you're getting whole grains. The first ingredient of a whole-grain food should say "whole," such as whole wheat, whole oats, whole rye flour, or whole barley.

4. Substitute unsaturated fats (good) for saturated fats (bad). All fats should be consumed with moderation, but some are better than others. Unsaturated fats can reduce your risk for heart disease by lowering total cholesterol and low density lipoprotein cholesterol (LDL), or "bad" cholesterol. Saturated and trans fats have the opposite effect on cholesterol. Saturated fats are found in meats, poultry and dairy products. Trans fats are present mostly in baked goods (such as crackers and cookies) and in fried foods (french fries and doughnuts, for example). The word "hydrogenated" on a package is a red flag that the food contains trans fat. The two main sources of unsaturated fats include monounsaturated fats, which are found in olive, peanut and canola oils, and polyunsaturated fats found in vegetable oils, such as safflower, corn and soy oils. Omega 3 fatty acids are also good sources of polyunsaturated fats found mostly in seafood, such as salmon, herring and cold-water fish, and in walnuts and flaxseeds. You can also find eggs and whole grain pastas and waffles enriched with Omega 3s. With the exception of Omega 3s, polyunsaturated fats should be used sparingly because they block the body's absorption of good cholesterol.

5. Drink water. On average, the body is 60 percent comprised of water. Water is essential to all bodily functions. It regulates body temperature, aids digestion, lubricates joints, flushes out waste and carries nutrients and oxygen to cells. We lose water every day through breathing, urine, perspiration and bowel movements, making it vital to replenish your body's water supply. How much water you need each day will depend on climate (in hot weather you'll need more), health status and activity levels. While the Institute of Medicine recommends approximately nine cups of water a day for women, a good rule of thumb is to drink enough water to avoid feeling thirsty. Thirst is usually a sign that you are not getting enough fluids. To stay hydrated, drink a glass of water with each meal and carry a water bottle with you throughout the day so you'll have water readily available when you need it.

6. *Supplement your diet.* Even with a healthy diet, most of us are unable to obtain all the vitamins and minerals we need from food alone. Dietary supplements help fill nutritional gaps and some even provide a protective effect against certain diseases. Supplements can't replace the benefits received from eating whole and nutritious foods, but are a good insurance policy for staying healthy. To supplement your diet, start taking a multivitamin daily. You should consider your age, health status and activity level when choosing a multivitamin. At the very least, it should meet the standard recommended daily allowances, especially for iron and calcium—two minerals that are essential for women's health. Look for the U.S. Pharmacopoeia (USP) sign on the label to assure that it meets quality and safety standards.

7. *Consider alternative protein sources.* When it comes to protein sources, most Americans rely far too much on meat and poultry. There are other great sources of protein, particularly plant-based sources, including beans, whole grains and nuts. For an alternative to cow's milk, consider soy or rice milk. Try eating more fish instead of meat and poultry. Additionally, choose healthier ways of cooking, such as baking, broiling and grilling instead of frying.

8. *Drink tea.* Although research is still being conducted on the benefits of tea, the high flavonoid (antioxidant) content in tea may reduce the risk of heart attack, stroke and cancer. Researchers have found that flavonoids—which are also found in red wine and dark chocolate—can lower cholesterol, prevent inflam-

mation and protect arteries from hardening. Green tea comes highly recommended as it is made from unfermented tea leaves and undergoes less processing, but black tea and other teas are also beneficial. Green tea is also lower in caffeine and has higher antioxidant properties. Herbal teas can also be great for treating insomnia, colds, cramps and a wide variety of other conditions.

Tea often contains caffeine, so be careful to drink it long before bedtime or choose a caffeine-free tea. Although green and black teas come in decaffeinated varieties, there is usually a small amount of caffeine that remains (usually about 5 percent)—a small caveat to keep in mind if you have sleep problems or want to avoid caffeine all together. You can enjoy tea cold or hot and enjoy the same benefits. If you normally drink coffee, try substituting tea instead. There are many varieties with robust and rich flavors that would satisfy the most discriminating coffee lover. In general, caffeine, like all other things, should be consumed in moderation. Caffeine can cause irritability, insomnia, heart palpitations and dizziness.

9. Allow for a few indulgences. Give yourself permission to indulge in the foods or snacks you love without guilt or shame. When possible, plan ahead and make adjustments in your diet. For instance, if you are going to have chocolate cake in the evening, cut back on the fat and sugar you consume during the day. If you can make your indulgence healthier, do so. Can you choose a low-fat or low-sugar option? Can you enjoy a smaller portion than normal? If you're a chocolate lover like me, choose dark chocolate with a high cocoa content—at least 60 percent—for heart health benefits. If you enjoy an occasional glass of wine or other alcoholic beverage, consider red wine. Like chocolate, red wine is high in flavonoids and is also great for heart health. Enjoy it in moderation. For women, the American Heart Association recommends no more than one drink per day. A drink is twelve ounces of beer, four ounces of wine, one and a half ounces of eighty-proof spirits or one ounce of one hundred-proof spirits. If you are trying to lose weight, are pregnant, or have diabetes, high blood pressure or another condition that may be adversely affected by alcohol, avoid wine and other alcoholic beverages all together.

discover the joy of movement

Physical activity is vital to our overall wellbeing. Its benefits go far beyond physical health. Movement unleashes our energy, liberates our spirits and opens our minds and bodies to new ways of being. How much we move our bodies is directly related to how we approach our lives. In the words of Aristotle, "We are what we repeatedly do." If we are rigid or physically tense, that rigidity and tension will be reflected in the choices we make in life. In contrast, when we are physically strong and supple, our life force flows through us freely and we are able to live with confidence and freedom.

Physical activity is so vital to our existence that no other health recommendation comes close to conferring the benefits that regular physical activity provides. Women who are physically active look and feel better, live longer and enjoy a better quality of life than sedentary women. Regular physical activity:

- Reduces the risk of dying of coronary heart disease—the number one killer of women

- Decreases the risk for stroke, colon cancer, diabetes, and high blood pressure

- Helps control weight

- Contributes to healthy bones, muscles, and joints

- Reduces falls among older adults

- Helps relieve the pain of arthritis

- Reduces symptoms of anxiety, depression and stress

- Promotes general health and is associated with fewer hospitalizations, physician visits, and medications

Despite all the health benefits, most of us aren't active enough to reap the benefits of regular physical activity. According to the Centers for Disease Control and Prevention (CDC), over half of U.S. adults aren't getting enough physical activity. In a recent survey by the American Heart Association, only 15 percent were willing to become more physically active to achieve their weight loss and health goals. The CDC recommends that adults engage in moderately intense physical activities (such as brisk walking, yoga or gardening) for at least thirty minutes on five or more days of the week or vigorously intense physical activity (such as jogging, aerobics or high-energy dancing) three or more days per week for at least twenty minutes per occasion.

the story of our lives is hidden in the way that we move

If you don't have a regular physical activity or exercise program, I will coach you (in the next few pages) on how to get started by taking small steps and breaking down the barriers that may be keeping you from experiencing the joy of movement. Remember, even a small increase in your activity level is helpful. No matter what your age or dress size—it is never too late to get started. Start slow and work your way up to either thirty minutes of moderate activity most days of the week or twenty minutes of vigorous activity three or more days a week.

break down the barriers to stay active

Now, you might be thinking that you don't have time to be active. Or you may be thinking that you hate exercise, "Never liked it, never will." I want you to let your guard down about being physically active so that you can see the many options available to you. There are many reasons why we women aren't as active as we should be. I was so fascinated by this issue that I decided to study it as part of my thesis for my master's degree. In the almost ten years since I initially surveyed a group of African American women professionals about their views on exercise, little has changed. The barriers to regular physical activity are universal, but they can be melted down.

1. Make physical activity a sacred exercise. Like all the practices and suggestions provided throughout this book, physical activity is about loving and knowing yourself in the deepest way possible. This depth of love and understanding of your true self—your spirit—is the foundation of your health and wellness. When performed with a conscious intention to build a body that is strong, light and healthy to carry your spirit, physical activity takes on a new dimension in your life. When you make physical activity a celebration of your life and spirit, an act of devotion and reverence to yourself and to God, exercise becomes a profound experience that you won't want to live without.

Movement is part of our nature. It brings harmony to every part of our being. When you exercise with mindful awareness of your movements, breath and thoughts, you will gain access to knowledge about yourself that you may not otherwise have access to. The parallel may not always be obvious, but exercise can teach us a lot about our strengths, weaknesses and overall approach to life. Life, like a yoga pose, can be challenging. Yet the breath is always available to guide us. The breath creates an opening within the body to move further or deeper into poses. Similarly, when we are challenged in life, sometimes all we need is a little breathing space to find the guidance and direction that we need to move forward. Maintaining a schedule of regular physical activity draws on and reveals our character and teaches discipline. It is the higher self that calls us to take better care of ourselves, to go out and walk, practice yoga or dance when we'd rather keep working or tending to the myriad of other things that pull and tug at us daily.

If you've ever been in the "zone" while exercising, then you know that it can be an elevating and meditative experience that awakens yet relaxes the mind and body. Studies have shown that exercise can induce alpha waves, which are a bridge between the conscious and subconscious in the brain. A close friend of mine notices that she has a heightened sense of intuition and clarity after about forty-five minutes of walking on the treadmill. She says that she finally came to grips with not being able to have children after a session on the treadmill. A mental picture of her being whole and complete, despite having a hysterectomy for fibroids, appeared that helped her see and accept a future that she had not previously envisioned.

Six Steps to Moving with Spirit

1. To begin to imbue your exercise with spirit, choose to exercise out of love for yourself rather than punishment for eating the wrong foods or out of hate for your body or weight. Practicing the exercises outlined in this and

other principles will help you cultivate this love if you don't have it right now. It may take some time to feel, but it is within you. It is the reason why you are reading this book. Deep down inside you know that you are being called to move and take better care of your body. Give yourself the breathing space you need to move and live in the grace and beauty of your body.

2. Begin your sessions with a prayer It can be as simple as, "Thank you for the ability to walk/practice yoga/dance/run." Or, take a deep breath to acknowledge that you are transitioning into a sacred time for health and healing.

3. Be conscious of what you are listening to while exercising. Make sure that it is soothing and uplifting to your mind, body and spirit. Many women enjoy working out to gospel or instrumental music. You may choose to forgo music all together. I find that some days music is great for my yoga practice and other times I need complete silence. When I go for walks outside, my music is the sound of birds chirping, trees swaying and the occasional sound of cars going by.

4. Be present while exercising. Your mind may wander, but gently bring it back by reminding yourself to focus on "right here and right now." A good way to stay present is to focus on your breath and movements, or a mantra or prayer.

5. Be open to receiving direction and guidance during or after your session.

6. Say another prayer of thanks at the end of your exercise session or lie or sit in silence for a few minutes and observe how you feel in your body.

2. Get past the time factor. By far, the most common excuse I hear women give for not exercising is "I don't have time." It's true; we are all busy and starved for time. Yet there is room somewhere in our daily schedule for exercise. Besides, for something as sacred and beneficial as exercise, it has to be one of our top priorities. I like to exercise first thing in the morning. It is part of my morning routine and sets the tone for my day. I find that when I don't get moving in the morning, I am less productive and alert. When I don't move in the morning, I usually end up stopping in the middle of the day to make up for what I missed.

Even a few minutes of movement throughout the day can make a big difference. So if you don't have a full thirty minutes to exercise all at one time, spread your exercise time throughout the day. Here's a simple plan to get you started:

- Be active for ten minutes in the morning before you go to work. Use this time to center and energize yourself for the day ahead.

- Walk for ten minutes after lunch. Walking aids digestion and is a great way to break away from the constant sitting most of us do during the workday.

- Devote another ten minutes to physical activity such as stretching when you return from work in the evening. It will help relieve the day's stress and prepare you for a good night's sleep.

There are so many other ways to "sneak" more activity into our daily lives. Here are a few simple and easy ways:

- Walk instead of driving whenever you can. When you do drive, park the car farther away than you normally would.

- Take the stairs instead of the elevator.

- Wash your car by hand.

- Walk your kids to school.

- Stretch when you wake up and before you go to bed.

- Dance, step in place, or do crunches while watching television.

3. Do something you enjoy. The surest way to stick to your exercise plan is by engaging in activities you love. If you aren't enjoying the activity the odds are slim that you'll keep doing it. If you're in pain or feel embarrassed or uncomfortable having other people around when you're exercising, your approach to staying fit will be overshadowed by dread instead of pleasure.

To find the right exercise, ask yourself, *What do I need out of my physical activity? Do I need to feel energized? Relaxed? Centered? Challenged? What conditions must be met to make it an enjoyable experience?* For many women, those conditions include:

Convenience: Is the studio or gym nearby? Is it something you can do at home or in your neighborhood with little or no props or equipment? Can you easily work it into your schedule with little disruption to your life? Keep things simple. The farther you have to travel and the more "stuff" you need, the less likely you are to stick with the activity.

Environment: Many women are uncomfortable in traditional gyms. What's your preference? Would you be more comfortable in a women's gym or fitness center or in the comfort of your home? Do you want to have other people around you (like a walking group) or do you prefer to be alone? Choose an activity compatible with the environment that you need to be fully engaged without feeling self-conscious or distracted.

Ability: Do you need specialized or advanced skills or abilities for the exercise? Be realistic about your abilities and choose activities that allow you to start where you are today but provide sufficient opportunities for you to challenge yourself and grow. It's noble to want to go out and run a charity marathon, but if you've been sedentary most of your life, walking might be the more suitable choice at first. You can always work your way up to jogging and eventually running.

If there's an activity that you always wanted to learn, look for an introductory class and work your way up. One of the reasons I fell in love with yoga was because I had to approach it with a beginner's mind—a complete departure from the way I normally approached things. Exercise teaches us that there are boundaries and limits to respect, including those of our bodies. Yet with practice, some of those limits can be dissolved. The era of "no pain, no gain" is gone. Be compassionate with yourself by respecting your abilities. In time, you will find joy and excitement in learning a new yoga pose, dance routine, or walking farther and faster than you have before.

You'll know you've found the right set of activities when you find yourself looking forward to doing them. If you haven't found that magical combination yet, try different types of exercise. The options are endless: yoga, Pilates, tai chi, swimming, dancing, running, kickboxing, walking, bicycling and more. The goal is to have at least two to three activities that will provide variety, enjoyment and challenge to your exercise program. Performing the same activity every day is the quickest way to boredom. Use your inner guide to determine which activity will best serve you on any given day. Some days, I need an hour of yoga. Other times, I awake feeling as if I am bursting with an energy that only free flow dancing will satisfy. At other times I need the meditative action of walking to center and balance me. Don't underestimate the power of your intuition to advise you on the best activity. If you usually walk but suddenly feel one day that you need to dance or run, give in to the impulse. Your intuition may be leading you toward an emotional release or breakthrough in some area of your life. Remember, our bodies

three keys to physical fitness

For a complete fitness program, include strength training and aerobic and flexibility exercises.

Aerobic exercise is any activity that uses large muscle groups in a continuous, rhythmic fashion for sustained periods of time. Walking, jogging, dancing and cardio workouts are all considered aerobic exercise.

Flexibility exercise is needed to maintain joint range of motion and reduce the risk of injury and muscle soreness. Always warm up before you stretch. Like strength conditioning, flexibility exercises should include stretching for all the major muscle groups.

Strength training includes exercises that have been shown to increase the strength of muscles, maintain bone health and improve balance, coordination, and mobility. Because strength training increases the rate of metabolism, it can also aid in weight loss and management. Calisthenics, free weights or machines are all muscle strengthening activities. Strength training becomes increasingly important as women age and should be a part of your physical activity program at least twice week.

Always check with your doctor before beginning any exercise program

are wise beyond what we consciously know. There is intelligence and memory in our muscles.

4. Don't let hair get in the way. When it comes to working out, worrying about ruining a nice hairdo is a real concern for many women, especially women of color. Looking your best is an important part of your overall wellness but shouldn't prevent you from staying fit. If you're avoiding exercise because you don't want to ruin your hair, consider styling your hair in ways that suit a more active lifestyle. Try a short haircut, pin curls, braids, twists or dreadlocks. Wraps, ponytails and straight hairstyles can also be a lot easier to maintain than styles that require a curling iron or large amounts of hairspray or other chemicals that might damage your hair.

Ideally, you wouldn't allow your hair to limit your activity choices, but it's a real choice that many of us make. The key is to find solutions and activities that help you strike a balance between your health and beauty needs. Remember, hair pins and clips are a tried and tested method for keeping hair in place. If you fear that humidity or being out in the sun will get to your hair, join a gym, try a workout tape or participate in other indoor activities. If you can't wash your hair after a sweaty workout, try a hair freshener that absorbs oils and neutralizes odors in the scalp. With patience and a little creativity, you'll learn how to sync your hair care demands with your active lifestyle so you can be both fit and fabulous.

5. Find support to stay motivated. Would you benefit from having a friend or a health coach to cheer you on? Having a support system to keep you motivated can pay off in big dividends. In just three months in our coaching program, some women lost as much as twenty pounds. After years of wanting to try tai chi, with the support of her health coach, one client finally decided to give it a try. We stressed the importance of social support in the program, and while some women found it hard to ask for help, others found support not only in their health coaches but also in family and friends. Mothers and daughters and sisters were working out together and enjoying a new way of bonding with each other. If you need help or support with your exercise or health goals, don't be afraid or embarrassed to ask for it. The most successful people all have a team to support them in specific areas of their lives. Why should you be any different? Asking for help is not a sign of weakness but the mark of a wise woman who knows when she needs a hand to reach newer heights. Sometimes just having the support of someone else is enough to give us the extra push we need to keep going. If you have a friend also trying to take better care of her health, why not team up? Take walks together or cheer each other on.

A health coach can provide expert guidance and support for not just achieving your current health goals but also for sustaining a healthy lifestyle by drawing on your own innate skills and abilities. A health coach will provide structure, accountability and motivation to help you realize your fullest potential and best health. You'll also learn new ways to use your inner resources to take action and stay motivated, not just in your health-related endeavors but in other areas of your life as well.

recharge and renew yourself with sleep

Nothing heals and replenishes us the way that sleep does. And nothing drags us down and wears us out like not getting enough. Sleep is the body's intuitive call for rest and renewal. As natural as day and night, sleep reminds us of the need to maintain balance between rest and activity. When we are exhausted and depleted, sleep refuels and recharges us for another day. When challenged with a difficult decision, we "sleep on it," knowing that a good night's sleep brings clarity and a fresh perspective.

Lack of sleep causes irritability, moodiness and depression. It impairs concentration and increases the risk of illness and weight gain. Losing sleep interferes with the production of hormones—including the ones regulating hunger, metabolism and libido. Chronic lack of sleep taxes the body and increases the presence of cortisol, a stress hormone associated with diabetes, hypertension and premature aging of the skin. Because most cell repair and regeneration of skin and muscles tissue takes place in the deeper stages of sleep, cheating ourselves out of a good night's rest can accelerate aging and make us look older than we really are.

Obtaining adequate sleep is a problem for women of all ages. Women are twice as likely to suffer from insomnia than men. So many things—such as caring for children, work, stress and hormones (menstruation, pregnancy and menopause)—affect our ability to sleep. Though there are ways to deal with it (such as working less and improving our sleep habits), we often cheat ourselves out of the vitality and health that comes with a good night's sleep. The truth is, far too many of us are accustomed to skimming on it. It's become a badge of courage and a sign of commitment to say that we "stayed up all night working" on a project. In our modern life, sleep is becoming more and more of a luxury. According to a National Sleep Foundation poll, half of the women said that sleep and exercise are the first things to be sacrificed when pressed for time. Time with friends and family, healthy eating and sex were the next things to go. Only 20 percent of women said that they'd work less when short on time or too sleepy!

Follow these tips for improving the quality and quantity of your sleep:

- *Stick to a regular schedule.* The body has an internal clock that tells us when to sleep and when to wake. Going to bed and waking up around the same time every day will keep you in tune with your sleep clock and set the stage for a happy sleep life. Try to get to sleep before midnight—preferably by 10 P.M. The hours before midnight, according to Ayurvedic philosophy, are the most restorative.

- *Call it a night.* Our minds often keep running long after our bodies have decided it's time to sleep. To get yourself in the frame of mind for sleeping, stop working a few hours before going to sleep. Use your journal to help you release repetitive thoughts and worries. When you catch yourself in bed worrying or thinking about what you need to do, gently tell yourself, "My work for the day is done." Beware of watching TV at night. Instead of relaxing you, watching TV can stimulate the mind and disrupt sleep.

- *Relax.* Establish a relaxation routine to help lull you to sleep. Take a warm bath. Essential oils, such as lavender and chamomile, are great for inducing sleep. Add a few drops to your bath water. You can also relax tense muscles by stretching or practicing progressive muscle relaxation. Avoid stimulating activities and substances like alcohol, nicotine and caffeine. Exercising is great and can even improve sleep but causes body temperature to rise, which can disturb your sleep. To be on the safe side, don't exercise three hours before bedtime. If you're prone to insomnia, avoid exercising five to six hours before bedtime.

- *Set the mood.* Sleep is a sensual experience. Engage your senses:

    Sight: Keep your bedroom clutter-free and visually pleasing. When you step into your bedroom, it should invite you to relax and release all your cares. Decorate your bedroom using colors, pictures and mementos that relax, invite and create a sense of harmony and tranquility. Turn the lights down as you prepare for sleep and turn them off when you're ready to turn in. Use an eye mask to block out light coming in from the street.

    Smell: Spray your room and linens with a light, aromatherapy spray containing calming scents like lavender, sandalwood, chamomile and neroli, or use scented candles and potpourri to keep the room smelling fresh. If you use an eye mask, spray it as well or use a scented one. I also like to massage lavender essential oil on my temples, behind my ears, and on the back of my neck.

    Touch: Start with a comfy mattress, then dress it with beautiful and soft linens and pillows. Wear relaxed, loose fitting clothes and keep the temperature cool or warm enough for you to be comfortable throughout the night.

    Sound: Turn the TV off as you prepare for sleep. Use soft music or silence to signal to your brain that you're transitioning into sleep mode. If you need background sound to go to sleep, try a white sound machine or music designed to induce sleep.

- *Get some sun.* Exposure to sunlight is key to regulating daily sleep patterns. Be sure to get outside every day (preferably in the morning) in natural sunlight for at least thirty minutes to reset your body's internal clock. Natural sunlight also helps to boost the production of vitamin D, eases depression and elevates mood. To get the most benefit from the sun, avoid wearing contact lenses and sunglasses while you're outdoors.

If you've tried all the aforementioned suggestions and still can't get enough sleep at night, try taking a nap. Naps boost brain power and energy. More and more companies are seeing the benefits of a good power nap and have designated areas in the office for a quick fifteen to twenty minute nap. Some people even secretly sneak a nap during the workday with their office door closed. If you can squeeze a nap in, try to get it in before 3 P.M. For some women, napping can make the problem worse. Napping too close to bedtime can also interfere with your normal sleep cycle. Lastly, if you have chronic sleep problems, seek help from a qualified health professional. It may be tempting to ask for a sleeping pill, but sleeping pills can make it harder to get to the root of sleep disorders. Ask for a complete exam and diagnosis, which may include a referral to a sleep center.

experience the healing power of touch

Touch is essential to our health and wellbeing. A gentle loving touch can reassure, heal and affirm us in ways that words never could. Touch is so vital that not getting enough of it can stunt our mental, emotional and physical growth and shorten our life. A traditional way of healing for centuries, the miracles Jesus performed were often through the healing power of touch. Egyptian tomb paintings depicted people being massaged, and the Chinese text *The Yellow Emperor's Classic of Internal Medicine*, dating back to 2700 B.C., recommends massage. Hippocrates, the father of Western medicine, advised a daily massage with oil after a bath for health maintenance.

Massage alleviates pain, reduces blood pressure, improves immune functioning, relieves muscle tension and accelerates wound healing and recovery. It also promotes the elimination of toxins and brings new life to tired and dull areas of the body by increasing circulation. Massage stimulates the production of feel-good hormones like oxytocin, which calms the mind and body. Dr. Kerstin Uväs-Moberg, author of *The Oxytocin Factor*, believes that oxytocin creates a sense of openness that may increase our intuitive abilities—like a mother knowing exactly what a baby wants. Intuition is one of those things that we tend to downplay, but if you've ever had an eerie feeling about someone or a situation, then later learned your gut feeling was right, you know intuition can save your life. The director of Behavioral Health at the Canyon Ranch—a popular health resort in Tucson, Arizona—says that people come away from the massage table with insights on how to approach the next phase of their lives, having such realizations as "I have to get out of my marriage" or "I've got to make a career change right now."

That exquisitely human contact we know as massage is in essence a universal birthright of our kind.

—RAPHAEL TUBURAN

Neuroscientists studying touch have found that there are small fibers on the skin that deal more with our unconscious and emotional selves than just our physical perception of being touched. The openness that massage and other types of bodywork facilitate, frees you to experience and release blocked emotions that may be affecting your health and your life. Many traditional cultures believe that trapped or imbalanced energy in the body is the precursor to illness and dys-function. Stress, trauma, illness and emotional pain can form layers of tension and pockets or knots of dis-ease that bring us out of balance. Restoring a healthy and balanced flow of energy through the body opens the door for optimal mental, physical, emotional and spiritual health. It strengthens, awakens and unleashes our vital energy.

Energy medicine has been gaining in popularity as more women discover the benefits of alternative and complementary approaches to health and healing. Reiki, the Japanese energy healing system, as well as other methods of healing touch can be found in hospitals around the country and are often provided by nurses. The National Institute of Health is funding studies of several energy-based healing systems including Reiki, acupuncture (based on Chinese meridians or rivers of energy), yoga and qigong. The studies are examining the effects of these healing modalities on a variety of health conditions, including heart disease, breast cancer, chronic back pain, HIV and osteoarthritis. Dr. Mehmet Oz, author and cardiac heart surgeon, introduced energy healing into the operating and recovery rooms at Columbia Presbyterian Medical Center in New York City over ten years ago. In a recent appearance on the Oprah Winfrey Show, Dr. Oz said, "We're beginning now to understand things that we know in our hearts are true but we could never measure. As we get better at understanding how little we know about the body, we begin to realize that the next big frontier in medicine is energy medicine. It's not the mechanistic part of the joints moving. It's not the chemistry of our body. It's understanding for the first time how energy influences how we feel."

You ought not to heal the body without the soul, for this is the great error of our day in treating the human body.

—PLATO

Find the right approach and practitioner. Along with the wonderful benefits of touch that I just described, the cumulative effects of modern life—which activate the stress response more often than any of us need—make massage, and other types of bodywork more of a necessity than a treat reserved for "special occasions." Our high-tech, low-contact world has so many of us starving to be touched. Time and distance makes the loving touch or embrace of friends and loved ones a rare commodity.

I find that nothing takes the place of healing more than going to a spa for a few hours or even an hour (or two) with my rolfer. Rolfing is a holistic bodywork method designed to realign the body with gravity by working soft tissue in a way that improves posture and helps the body work more efficiently. If you prefer a light touch with oil, then rolfing isn't for you. It can be painful, but worth it if you have chronic muscle aches and tension that don't respond to the average massage.

Before you set an appointment for a massage, decide which therapeutic approach will be best for you. Will the light touch of a Swedish massage, the heated stones used during a hot stone massage or the intense and focused pressure of deep tissue massage meet your needs? Do you need a method based on a system of energy balancing and healing? There is a wide range of techniques from Egyptian, Native American, Tibetan and Japanese energy healing traditions.

Do your research to find a method and practitioner that you're comfortable with.

A good massage therapist or bodyworker can read the language of your body without you ever having to say what hurts or aches. My rolfer just looks at the way I walk and carry myself and knows where the tension is in my body. Each place he massages, strokes and kneads tells a story. Often times, I am brought to tears. Other times, I am reminded of how hard I have been pushing myself. But every time, I end the session with him, grateful for the healing experience. My rolfer is a wise and kind Japanese man who gently offers instructions on how to better hold my body so that it works and moves more efficiently. But there is always a hidden message in his instructions that has to do more with how I approach life. *Let go...breathe...stand tall...let your arms sway.*

Sure, massage or visits to the spa can be indulgent and pampering, but I believe they are a necessary part of a modern woman's wellness strategy. A massage or other type of bodywork once a month is ideal. If you can't afford to pay for services, ask a spouse or partner, family member (even your kids) or friend for a massage. In our society we often associate touch with sex, but we know that touch more often has to do with the intangible, non-physical aspects of ourselves.

Giving and receiving a massage can be a healing experience for both the recipient and the giver. Our hands are an extension of our hearts. We can express and share the love and care in our hearts with just the simple act of touch. When we touch with loving and healing intention, our hands become powerful instruments of change and renewal.

Practice self-massage. When you can't benefit from the touch of someone else, give yourself massages. The gentle and loving touch of your own hand across your body is a wonderful way to deepen your connection with yourself. Ayurveda recommends self-massage every morning before a shower. This can be an extremely worthwhile self-care ritual if you have the time. When performed mindfully, self-massage, like other massages, allows you to fully inhabit your body and is a great way to center yourself. Self-massage fosters a positive intimacy with yourself that honors and celebrates your beauty. Learning and lovingly stroking every part of your body heightens your sense of self and builds confidence. The time you spend honoring yourself will fill you with a love and appreciation that will spill over into your relationships and other parts of your life. By practicing self-massage regularly, you'll also come to know your body and better recognize what is normal and when something might be awry.

To enhance your self-massage ritual, you may want to consider the many self-care products on the market including massage oils, rollers, balls and sticks. These products help to loosen the knots in the body and keep the energy flowing by increasing circulation. I use a very simple and low-cost technique that I learned from a back specialist to get the most out of self-massaging:

- Take two tennis balls and place them in a long sock.

- Tie a knot in the sock to prevent the balls from rolling out of the sock.

- Lie on the floor and place the balls in the area that needs massaging.

- Roll your body or body part gently against the balls. Try applying steady pressure instead of rolling your body for deeper relaxation of the muscle.

This technique works wonders and is a life-saver if you have arthritis in your hands or find massaging with your hands to be tiring.

Learn to balance your energy. You can also learn how to balance energy yourself. Yoga works with the subtle energies in the body. When I don't do my routine of Sun Salutations in the morning, I drag around and feel less energetic. It's an instant energy booster I can't do without. There are also many other resources, including books and classes on how to use color, crystals, chanting and other aides to balance energy. Look for classes in Reiki, healing touch, tai chi or other energy-based wellness systems in your area. On your path, keep an open mind, empower yourself with information and use your intuition to guide you to the tools that will best work for you.

Each patient carries his own doctor inside him. They come to us not knowing that truth. We are our best when we give the doctor who resides within each patient a chance to go to work.

— ALBERT SCHWEITZER, M.D.

take charge of your health

Honoring your body includes remembering to schedule regular preventative check-ups and screenings, including:

- **General Health:** Physical exam once a year.

- **Heart Health:** Blood pressure at least every two years. Cholesterol at age twenty—discuss with your doctor or nurse about frequency thereafter.

- **Bone Health:** Discuss with your doctor at age forty.

- **Diabetes:** Blood glucose test once a year.

- **Breast Health:** Mammogram every one to two years, starting at age forty. Monthly breast self-exams beginning at age twenty. A clinical breast exam should be performed during routine gynecological visits.

- **Reproductive Health:** Pap test and pelvic exams every one to three years. Sexually Transmitted Diseases (STD) tests before initiating sexual intercourse.

- **Colorectal Health:** Yearly, beginning at age fifty.

- **Eye and Ear Health:** Whenever you notice any visual or hearing problems, or at least one exam from twenty to twenty-nine years of age, at least two exams from ages thirty to thirty-nine, and every two to four years at age forty and thereafter.

- **Skin Health:** Monthly mole self-exam, including an exam by a doctor every three years starting at age twenty.

- **Oral Health:** Dental exam one to two times every year.

During your visit to any health care provider, ask questions about anything you don't understand. If you're diagnosed with a health condition, empower yourself with information so that you and your doctor can make the best decisions on the course of treatment.

To make the most of your doctor's visit, the National Women's Health

Information Center suggests the following:

- **Write your questions and concerns.** Before your appointment, make a list of what you want to ask. When you're in the waiting room, review your list and organize your thoughts. You can share the list with your doctor or nurse.

- **Give your doctor a list of your medications.** Mention what prescription drugs and over-the-counter medicines, vitamins, herbal products, and other supplements you're taking.

- **Be honest about your diet, physical activity, smoking, alcohol or drug use, and sexual history.** Not sharing information with your doctor or nurse can be harmful!

- **Talk about sensitive topics.** Your doctor or nurse has probably heard it before! Don't leave something out because you're worried about taking up too much time. Be sure to talk about all of your concerns before you leave.

- **Ask questions about any tests and your test results.** Get instructions on what you need to do to get ready for the test(s) and if there are any dangers or side effects. Ask how long it will take to get the results.

- **Ask questions about your condition or illness.** If you are diagnosed with a condition, ask your doctor how you can learn more about it. What caused it? Is it permanent? What can you do to help yourself feel better? How can it be treated?

- **Ask your doctor about any treatments he or she recommends.** Be sure to ask about all of your options for treatment. Ask how long the treatment will last and if it has any side effects.

- **Ask your doctor about any medicines he or she prescribes for you.** Make sure you understand how to take your medicine. What should you do if you miss a dose? Are there any foods, drugs, or activities you should avoid when taking the medicine? Is there a generic brand of the drug you can use?

- **Ask more questions if you don't understand something.** If you're not clear about what your doctor or nurse is asking you to do or why, ask to have it explained again.

If you're uncomfortable with the doctor's bedside manner, get another doctor. Your uneasiness can affect your willingness to be open and honest about what's ailing you. Know that women and men are often treated differently by doctors, and our physical complaints are often dismissed as "hysteria."

You live in your body every day. You are the expert on your body. I know of a woman who says she first learned that she had ovarian cancer from a dream. If something prompts you to schedule a doctor's appointment, honor that voice. Seek a second and a third opinion if necessary. Use your intuition along with the information that you have collected about your health condition and your health care provider's advice to make the choice that's best for you.

Regularly practicing the body awareness exercises and the wellness solutions outlined in this book will help you attend and attune to your body in a way that heightens your sensitivity to your mental, emotional, spiritual and physical needs. Love and listen to your body. It is wiser than any of us knows.

principle six

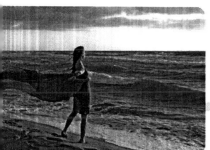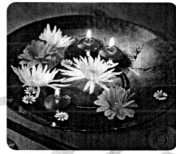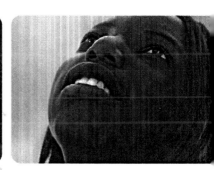

live in beauty

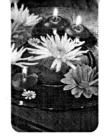

Hozho is a Navaho term often expressed as "walking in beauty." There is no direct English translation for the word, but it encapsulates the idea of harmony, beauty, balance, health and wellbeing. It is a state of being and a way of living. The Navaho approach to life is to live a long life in hozho. To me, this is the essence of wellness. To continually seek, live and be in health, peace and balance with myself, others and the environment. Quite simply, hozho is the good life, that *joie de vivre*, the joy in feeling connected to and part of a greater universe that is beautiful and good.

There is a lot in this world to get down about. But if we choose to see past the hurt and disappointments, we can't deny that there is beauty everywhere. It's in the trees, music, art, food, people and places we love. The more we immerse ourselves in it, the more our own natural beauty shines through.

Recognizing that we are all beautiful is a good starting point to living in beauty. We often hesitate to describe ourselves as beautiful. We don't fit the mold. But physical beauty is just one aspect of beauty. Inner beauty is everlasting. It's not a consolation prize for not having a "great" body, it is the prize. Yet knowing that doesn't discount the value of sprucing up our looks. Our early foremothers knew the power of painted fingernails and rouge on the lips to not only lift a woman's spirit, but the spirits of others around her.

It's the beauty within us that makes it possible for us to recognize the beauty around us.

— JOAN CHITTISTER

choose to see and be beauty

Beauty is more than skin deep. Beauty is a quality that radiates from us when we are living in health and in harmony with our innermost self. Beauty is like our cells. It is the stuff that we are made of. It is in each and every one of us. There is beauty in every step of our creation. There is a beautiful miracle that happens every time someone is conceived. The delight of one lucky sperm to meet an egg. Then from that one chance encounter an incredible set of events conspire, leading to the culmination of that fateful event: your birth.

I grew up thinking I was ugly. Now that I know that I was actually very beautiful, I've gotten old. Old is not ugly, it's just not the beautiful I use to be when I didn't know I was. Now I know that true beauty is spiritual and with it comes a peace that brings a healthy expression of self.

—ALFREDA, AGE 57

Now that's a very simplified version of the whole process. But it is a reminder that we are born of beauty. Beauty is within us. Always. And the more we cultivate it by the many things that we do to be whole and well, the more beautiful we become. The more it radiates from us.

We seek beauty both on the inside and out because we know beauty inherently. We remember beauty. We are beauty.

As women, we can't live without mirrors because even when we're unable to consciously see our own beauty, a part of us still knows

ten ways to bring out your natural beauty

Schedule a visit to a salon or spa for beauty treatments. *Take* a bath with bubbles or skin-nourishing oils once a week. *Surround* yourself with colors, things and people that bring out your beauty. *Journal* about the qualities that make you beautiful. *Dance* naked in your living room. *Do* something nice for someone else. *Take* a walk. *Make* sleep a priority. *Treat* your skin with nourishing and gentle products. *Wear* your favorite fragrance.

that we are beautiful, regardless of what our physical attributes may be. Sure, we want to make sure that there isn't toilet paper hanging off the back of our skirts, but our fascination with our reflection goes deeper than that. Mirrors have long been used as metaphors for truth and personal growth. When we look in mirrors, we are looking for more than lipstick stains on our lips. Ultimately, we want our beauty to shine without obstructions. Worrying about hair being out of place or food in our teeth can also be a metaphor for the inner work that we are doing to clear our path to wellness. What we look like on the outside does matter. I'm not talking about being perfect or fussing over our looks, but honoring the beauty inside by allowing it to shine on the outside.

The colors that we choose to wear and the outfits that we put together can energize us and the people around us. Colors are powerful vehicles of communication. The colors we choose can be potent symbols and motivators. I love the color red because it is a powerful color. Red makes a statement, and I feel vibrant when I am wearing it. My journal is red, and I keep words of inspiration around my desk in red ink. Red conjures up so many positive and affirming qualities for women. Red is attention-grabbing. A red dress has become the symbol of heart disease awareness among women. Women of the Red Hat Society wear red hats to celebrate their maturity. Interestingly, Native Americans walk a red road toward wholeness, truth and balance.

Our beauty is a gift we share with the world. I once came across a model's website where she declared that her mission was to inspire the world with beauty. I found her declaration intriguing. I never thought of physical beauty in that way, yet it made perfect sense to me. Here was a physically beautiful woman who recognized her beauty and declared that she was going to use it to inspire others. That's powerful. We can all be shining examples of beauty in our own unique way.

I've admired the beauty of other women, and it has inspired me to bring out my own beauty. Likewise, I've received compliments about the way I've worn my hair, applied make-up or on a pair of shoes. These everyday "acts of beauty" can inspire other women to try new things to enhance their own beauty. Take for instance the cashier who used to work at the drug store near my home. She would often admire my make-up. One day while cashing me out, she told me she was wearing the foundation I suggested and that she thought of me as she applied her make-up that morning. It touched my heart. I complimented her on how beautiful she looked (and she did). I could tell that it meant a lot to receive my approval. Looking back, I never set out to do anything but go into that store and get the supplies I needed. This memory reminds me that we never know how deeply we are touching people, simply by being ourselves. Honoring the many ways that beauty expresses itself in us and in other women is a form of gratitude, a way of acknowledging the profound goodness and grace that resides in each of us.

Taking joy in life is a woman's best cosmetic

—ROSALIND RUSSELL

One of the most inspiring and beautiful women I know is my grand-mother—gray hair, mumu dress and all. At seventy-eight years old, she isn't as energetic as she used to be and suffers from diabetes. But she has an incredible glow, a beauty and peace emanating from her that I find incredibly soothing and comforting. Her beauty is a result of a well-lived life. She hasn't traveled the world or eaten at fancy restaurants, but she has a sense of self and Spirit that attracts love. She has an unshakeable faith and a heart of gold. In her younger days, she had a pioneering spirit and a larger vision for her family that I am now reaping the benefits of through the many opportunities available in this country.

For years, my mother was in the beauty business. She owned a beauty salon and her own cosmetics line. As a girl growing up, my sisters and I would take turns working in the salon on weekends when it got busy. I didn't make the connection back then, but being at the salon, helping to transform women, set the stage for my work in life. There is something special about having someone do your hair or paint your toenails. It is healing.

The documentary film *Beauty Academy of Kabul* tells the story of American hairdressers who travel to the capital of Afghanistan to open a school to teach women how to style hair and apply make-up. Under the Taliban's oppressive regime, women were not allowed to work outside of their homes. Beauty salons were banned and women were forced to cover themselves up from head to toe. But interestingly, women secretly ran beauty salons in their homes and their cus-tomers would sneak off to patronize them. One of the most touching aspects of the film was seeing all the women who desperately wanted to attend the school. It was an opportunity to earn a living and help their families. Watching the film brought tears to my eyes as I imagined my mother coming to the United States in need of making a new life in a foreign country. I was also struck by one of the American hairdressers who saw the role of the Afghan women being trained as healers. If there is one thing connecting all women, it is that desire to express our beauty. Our identity is often tied to our hair. We make statements by the way we wear our hair and the clothes we choose to wear. That avenue of self-expression was taken away from Afghani women, and the hairdressers, in their own way, were trying to help the women regain their sense of freedom and dignity.

This world is nothing more than Beauty's chance to show Herself. And what are we? — Nothing more than Beauty's chance to see Herself. For if Beauty were not seeking Herself, we would not exist.

—GHALIB

step into the beauty of the world

Stepping out into the world through travel can be an incredibly freeing act. Travel can free us from everyday routines and transport us to different places, allowing us to learn about and experience other people, cultures, music and food. Through our travels, we can gain a fresh perspective on life if we open our minds and hearts to the new people and things around us. Travel journalist Pico Iyer says it best in his famed essay, "Why We Travel": the beauty of travel is the fresh perspectives that we as travelers bring to the people we encounter. "You can teach them what they have to celebrate as much as you celebrate what they have to teach," Iyer asserts.

Traveling can also reaffirm your life, giving you a deeper appreciation for the people and everyday routines you left behind.

Last year, returning from an extraordinary visit to Venezuela, I returned with a greater awareness of what traveling could do not just for me but also for the places and people that I visited. It was my first time in South America, and I was excited. I had recently compiled my personal passion list—a list of fifty things that I love (and need to do or enjoy more). Travel was number one on the list. While I traveled fairly often on business, it had been a while since I traveled outside the country. I wanted a completely different experience from my everyday life—and that's exactly what I got. I was traveling solo, but not alone, though I did not know any of the people that I would be spending the next ten days with. As part of a delegation of eighteen people organized by Global Exchange, we were in Venezuela on a "reality tour" to learn about Afro-Venezuelan culture and the political and social changes occurring in the country.

We were a group of open-mined people from all walks off life: white, black, Latino; teachers, a student, a private detective and university professors.We traveled to Caracas and small towns in the Barlovento region—an area near the Caribbean coast that rarely shows up on Venezuelan maps. But Barlovento is an important cultural mecca in Venezuela. It is the area where the majority of Afro-Venezuelans lives and celebrates the annual Fiesta de San Juan.

We spent six days in Barlovento, where a local family prepared the majority of our meals. I have to admit, when I first heard that we would be eating at the same place for nearly a week, I was concerned. Liliana, the wife of one of the community leaders, would be doing all the cooking. *I hope she can cook!* I thought to myself. But the first night we had dinner at Liliana's, all my concerns vanished.

Each day was a lesson in letting go and accepting things as they are, including the fact that little creatures, such as a small frog, might appear in my hotel bathroom. Oddly enough, the frog made an appearance the first and last night of my stay in Barlovento. I wondered if it was trying to send me a message. The heat was sweltering and by the third day, I realized that applying make-up was futile. Each day I started wearing less and less, as if I was shedding my American pretenses. Yet, I felt incredibly free and beautiful (though sweaty!).

At Liliana's one afternoon, we discovered *tetas*, frozen fruit treats that are shaped like breasts. Tetas spark a number of jokes that might otherwise be considered inappropriate in the United States, but Venezuelans—especially Barloventeños, we're told, don't have the same hang-ups that we Americans have about our bodies. The difference is noticeable. Women of all shapes and sizes walk confidently and gracefully as they go about their day.

During our stay in the region, we visited several *cumbes*—communities established by freed and escaped slaves. We visited schools, a women's sewing cooperative, a community clinic ran by a Cuban doctor, several political and community groups, and attended the San Juan Cultural festival in Curiepe. Curiepe was founded by former slaves in the early 1700s. Although the festival is celebrated throughout the country, the Curiepe festival is the largest, attracting people from around the country, and is not just a veneration of St. John the Baptist. It is more of a celebration of Afro-Venezuelan culture. Everywhere we went, people opened up their arms and homes to us, allowing us to learn more about their lives, their struggles, and their dreams. In the cumbes, children fascinated by foreigners would follow as we toured their community. Throughout our meetings and encounters, we asked a lot of questions, oftentimes questions that our hosts could not respond to. But some of our questions made the locals think and look at their work in a new way. At the women's cooperative, where they were working on a large order of uniforms for the communications ministry, questions were asked about the cooperative movement and free trade. Our host had not seen herself as part of a larger movement but she said our questions sparked a desire in her to know more about the cooperative initiative in the country. We had a similar experience at Mango d' Occay, a cumbe where an organic cocoa processing plant is being built by the government. The plant will be operated by a cooperative that is being organized in the community, providing a source of employment and income for residents in the area. One of the leaders of the co-op, after speaking with us outside where cocoa and other plants are being grown in the community, said that she never thought that what she was doing with the co-op was helping people, and our visit gave her work more meaning.

Back from Venezuela, I am still appreciating what I learned there and the opportunity to not just be a tourist but also a traveler fully engaged with the culture and people. There is a strong connection to the earth and nature there. When I eat now, I often think about and give thanks for all the people who had a role in bringing the food that I am enjoying to my plate. This is a remnant of seeing the lake where the fish we ate while in Barlovento came from and drinking freshly squeezed passion fruit, guyabana and other fruit juices that Liliana and her family would serve with each meal. Being reminded how other people out-side of the United States are so much more connected to the land, I am more conscious about the environment and the source of our food here. I am more appreciative of the abundance and convenience of the food available to me.

While riding on our tour bus through the trees and mountains, with indigenous music playing in the background, at times I'd be swept away in the moment by the beauty of what I was seeing, hearing and experiencing. There are so many small encounters, discussions, attempts to communicate, bits of humor lost in translation and other nuances that colored and shaped the trip. Yet despite the great experience, by day ten I wanted to come home. The evening I returned, I sat in my living room with a friend, detailing memories and displaying mementos from my trip. I was beaming. "Show and tell," he called it. I played music from Barlovento, danced, sang, reviving the infectious energy of Curiepe in my living room. I look back at the excitement and enthusiasm I had in the days following my return from Venezuela, and I can't remember anything since—besides writing this book—that so excited and ignited me.

Life is either a daring adventure or nothing.

—HELEN KELLER

Is it time to start planning a getaway, spiritual retreat or adventure tour to revive your spirit and expand your worldview? A day trip, a small town thirty miles away, can offer us a journey of learning or relaxation. I often go on getaways by myself—spending two or three days in a place I've never visited, in small towns like Richmond or Williamsburg. America is distinctive in that so many other cultures make up the fabric of our country, and a new cultural experience is only a car, plane or bus ride away. Of course, there is nothing like traveling to a foreign country where you are compelled to step outside of yourself, your language and your luxuries. But both domestic and international travel has a lot offer.

If you haven't traveled in a while or you've yet to visit the place of your dreams, what would bring you closer to that place? What can you begin to do to plan the trip? What about building a treasure map or visualizing what it will be like for you to be enjoying and basking in your dream destination? What are you doing? Are you being pampered? Sitting on the beach? Or learning about local culture and history? Consider starting a travel fund or committing to a date to take the trip. In the meantime, look for opportunities to travel, if not only in your mind or a few blocks away. Try visiting a museum that celebrates or memorializes the culture and the people you long to meet. Visit a restaurant; learn the dances or language indigenous to the area; or try cooking the food. Doing these things can enrich your everyday life and make your actual visit richer and more colorful.

make your home a sanctuary

Home is where the heart is. Our homes are unique environments, reflecting our personalities, passions, lifestyles, memories and possessions. Sometimes all that we have, materially-speaking, is in our homes. Our homes represent our dreams. They remind us of where we've been and where we want to go.

Our homes should be sanctuaries, places where we rest when we are tired, where we rejuvenate, breathe and live freely. After a long day at the office, running errands or traveling, there's nothing like coming home. The familiarity of our surroundings, the favorite couch, pillow or room can have a comforting and relaxing effect that cannot be duplicated anywhere else. The feeling of being home, not just in a physical space, but within oneself, is cause for celebration. Often times, lying in my bedroom or on the couch in my living room, feeling completely relaxed, at home and at peace, I say to myself, "This is the life." You don't have to live in a big or fancy home to feel like you're living large. In fact, many people are downsizing their homes, opting for the freedom, simplicity and lower costs that come with living in a smaller home. In a big or small place, we can gain a sense of expansiveness simply by creating space in our homes and lives to appreciate the beauty within and around us.

An orderly home—not necessarily pristine, just clutter free—allows us to live more freely and openly. Order lets us move about our spaces unobstructed by the reminders of daily life—like piles of clothes that need to be washed, unopened mail and toys that need to be put away.

We can think more clearly and see things as they really are when things are in their place. I once had a professional organizer come over to help me organize my home office. The one thing she left with me was the concept that everything has a place. Oftentimes, the items I couldn't find a place for were things I didn't need. In that case, I was to either throw them out or donate them. A sanctuary is not filled with things that we have no use for. But rather, it is filled with things and people that make our lives more comfortable and meaningful.

Small changes to a space have a huge impact. Couples can completely change their sex lives by redecorating or rearranging their bedrooms, and families can grow closer by creating spaces that make it easy and comfortable for family members to commune. A room that is airy and bright as opposed to cluttered and dark can lift our spirits and give us the breathing space we need to relax, gather or create. Personally, I find it easier to work at home when my desk is clear. But I do most of my writing in my living room, where I have more open space, more natural light and am surrounded by what I love, such as candles, silk pillows and chenille throws.

Our internal and external environments feed off each other. What we experience internally expands outwardly. Likewise, what we see and feel around us can affect our thoughts, emotions and health. Our home environment can stifle or promote our well being.

Do you feel stifled or uninspired in your home? What kind of energy or feeling do you wish to invite in your home? You can make the best of where you are right now by creating a sanctuary that honors your personal taste and lifestyle. There are many simple, cost-effective ways to transform your home into the haven you deserve. The good thing is that you don't have to move into a new place, buy new furniture or spend an exorbitant amount of money.

Try the simple steps below to beautify your home:

- **Surround yourself with things that you love.** Artwork and other crafts you create or buy bring creativity and beauty into your space. But don't bring things into your home that you don't like. If you can get what you want, you should. There is nothing like getting something you really don't like because it was cheaper and you now have to look at it every day.

- **Color your world.** Is it time to refresh your home environment with new colors and textures? Don't tie yourself to your existing color scheme. Bring in pillows in your favorite material or colors. Chenille and silk fabrics add a sense of luxury, warmth and comfort. Try painting the walls a new color to reflect the energy or mood you would like to create in different rooms.

- **Use candles to create a Zen-spa-like atmosphere.** Candles provide an easy and affordable way of decorating and adding ambiance, color, light and warmth to your home. Aromatherapy candles can help you create just the right mood. Try lavender to help you sleep or vanilla for warmth and comfort.

- **De-clutter your home.** As part of your new commitment to wellness, go through your home and throw out or donate things that are no longer part of the new lifestyle you're creating. If you're reluctant to do this, start out slowly. Go through each room of your home and find one item that you need to discard or clean. Go through the mail and piles of paper you have been pushing off. Sorting through piles of paper can be time consuming, so you may have to take this in small chunks. But the key is to get started. As you sort, determine which documents you still need, what can be thrown away, what requires action (a follow up call, for example) and what should be filed. If you don't have a filing system, set one up. Major categories might include: Bills, Health, Home, Warranties, Computer, Kids and Finances.

  Is it time to clean the curtains or drapes, mop the floor or clear out the medicine cabinet? Commit to taking on one room at a time. You might be surprised how much you enjoy this process. Getting rid of objects that take up space in your home is liberating. It may inspire you to let go of other stuff that no longer serves or enhances your life.

- **Open the windows.** According to some estimates, we spend 90 percent of our lives indoors. Indoor pollution can be a real problem. In fact it is one of the top five environmental health risks. Chemicals sprayed in the home such as household cleaners or hair products and those that are released by certain paints and household goods are just a few of the many potential sources of indoor air pollutants. Allow fresh air to flow through and natural light to brighten your home by opening windows, blinds and curtains.

- **Keep flowers and plants in your home.** Flowers and plants add beauty and life to a home. Plants also help to purify the air and can remove certain harmful chemicals such as benzene (found in most household cleaning agents) and formaldehyde (present in paper products including grocery bags, paper towels and foam insulation). For the most benefit, have a plant for approximately every ten square yards of floor space, that's about two to three plants for the average living room with an eight or nine foot ceiling (you'll need more plants if your ceilings are higher). Peace lily, gerbera daisies, bamboo palm, English ivy, and mums and are among the top plants for improving indoor air quality, according to studies led by NASA.

- **Create a get-away room.** Your get-away room is where you can completely relax; it is uncluttered, and elegantly simple. Keep the things that you need to help you relax there, such as music, books, candles, flowers, and pictures of loved ones. If you can't commit one room for this, find a corner or nook in a room and make it your sacred space. It could be an armchair near a window with a small table next to it where you sip tea, read inspirational books, meditate or just sit in silence. You might also keep pictures or objects that remind you of your goals, such as a treasure map or vision board, a photo of a tranquil place that you have visited or long to visit. Whatever draws you inward, nurtures and soothes your spirit and gets you back in touch with yourself is appropriate. If you have kids or live with others, ask them to respect your sacred space. You set the ground rules. Is anyone else allowed to enter that space? What can or can't they do or say when they are there? Is there a way that you can block it off if it's in a corner with a curtain or room divider, for example? Devoting a special place for reflection, dreaming, contemplation and meditation elevates your commitment to wellness and personal growth to a higher level. The more you spend time in your sacred space, the more you will want to be there. And the more that you are there experiencing tranquility and beauty, the more your life will reflect these qualities.

define your (life) style: putting it all together

Style is expression. It is an expression of our spirit, our true selves—our essence. Style is how we approach things, our methods, our passions expressed through the many aspects of life. Most of us associate style with fashion and beauty. While important, these are just two pieces of the tapestry that make up a lifestyle—the approach or philosophy upon which we base many of our choices and actions.

A lifestyle is how we choose to define, design and live our lives. What is your *life style*? When we are forced to follow or adopt someone else's style, we often feel stifled and inauthentic. When you embrace a life that allows you free expression of your spirit, you can create a lifestyle that reflects your personality, needs, desires and values. Your lifestyle is intimately connected to how you view life, the world and your experience in it. For example, if you believe that you should be feasting at life, soaking in and enjoying as much as possible, you will be driven to act in accordance with this value, which may take you around the world, experiencing exotic lands, music and food.

In the health arena, we spend a lot of time telling people that it's all about lifestyle choices, and it is. But we often fail to convince people to change their behaviors because we are imposing on them a particular view of life that may not be their own. We are all unique individuals, and our styles reflect that individuality.

For each of us, facts, figures, advice and recommendations have to resonate with us, striking a tune that rings true in our hearts. Yes, we all know that we have to eat better and exercise more. But what does it mean to you? If your approach to life is one of no limitations or restrictions, the suggestion that you must conform to a strict diet that prevents you from eating the foods you enjoy will have you running for the nearest exit. Now, I do believe we should eat foods that we enjoy. Our lifestyle should allow us to do this without compromising our commitment to good health. Once you are in tune with your heart's true desires—and hopefully good health is one of them—your style or approach to life will begin to reflect that value. We have to define our lives for ourselves, being open to the wisdom of our inner voices and the voices of others. Our lifestyle may evolve as we age, mature, learn and grow with experience. But it should always allow room for change and expansion. Without a willingness to step outside the box or the routine of the everyday, life gets dull and boring. It should also allow us to seek help when we need it, admit weakness while strengthening our resolve, enjoy life's pleasures and act in ways that best express who we are.

Revisit your picture of wellness. At the beginning of this book, you created a vision of wellness. Has that picture changed? Is your vision true to your inner beauty and power? Is it open and expansive? If it isn't, I encourage you to recreate that picture right now, taking into consideration the new insights that you may have gained about yourself from the suggestions, practices, questions and exercises in this book. Play with the vision you created, adding more color and detail. Let your imagination run wild. Create your life of wellness from a bigger and larger vision and commit to living from that place of expansion, opportunity and beauty.

Thomas Moore notes in his book *Dark Nights of the Soul*, "Beauty takes you out of your cramped, merely personal worries and sets you down in a field of eternity. The essence of spirituality is an enlargement of vision. The experience may only last a moment, but in these matters a moment is enough. You need a transcendent sense of things, not one that lets you escape from your situation, but one that gives you an added perspective." Moore reminds us that even a glimpse of beauty can change us. It can inspire us. And sometimes that's all we need, a little inspiration to see the bigger picture or to see something in ourselves and others that we had not noticed before. When we live in beauty, we live from an attitude of openness and receptivity instead of restriction and denial.

As you design your life to reflect your values about health and wellness, consider the following questions: Are you approaching life with an open mind and heart? Are you living a life true to your values? If not, how can you begin to start living your values today? Does your worldview and lifestyle allow you to celebrate and appreciate the beauty in and around you? How can you bring more beauty and joy into your life? What can you start doing today to bring you closer to the ultimate reality that you are creating for yourself? It doesn't have to be big. Just do *something* to start affirming your picture of wellness. Take a walk. Block off some quiet time for yourself or do some research on a topic that has piqued your interest. Make the connection with each step you take. Choose to see each step as part of a deliberate and intentional action designed to create the healthy, beautiful and balanced life you desire. The vision, affirmations and actions are part of the plan and practice of aligning your life energy with your values and goals.

Set concrete goals. If you haven't set concrete goals, take the time to do that now. Lay the cards out on the table. What is realistic for you right now? Trying to make sweeping changes all at once is a recipe for failure and disappointment. What key areas of wellness (mind, body, heart and spirit) do you think you need to start making a priority? What will be the springboard for you? What area do you think will create the opening in your mind and life so that you can take the next leap and move fully into a life of wellness?

As you take action to bring your vision to life, how will you stay motivated? Who will make up your support team? How will you draw on your inner resources to generate positive energy, motivation and thoughts to stay in the game? Even the most mundane and seemingly unrelated things can be connected to your vision and inspire you to move forward. The pair of sneakers that you wear on your walk can be a symbol of your unique path. The trip to the supermarket can be infused with the spirit and knowledge that you are going in to purchase and enjoy the bounty of the earth. This might sound a little nebulous, but for me walking into the Whole Foods store in my neighborhood gives me this feeling of, "Wow!" The first section I see walking in is the produce section, which excites me with all the luscious colors and aromas of fresh fruits and vegetables. They may have intentionally set it up that way, perhaps to get me to spend more. But, I know that when I walk into that store, my energy shifts up. I feel good when I walk out, and I feel like I'm doing something good for myself.

Go confidently in the direction of your dreams and live the life you've imagined.

—HENRY DAVID THOREAU

Know that it's never too late. We live in a limitless universe. Our challenge is to consciously accept and live in alignment with that truth. Now is the time to live large, bold and true, fully embracing the wonderful possibilities for your life. It's never too late, and you are never too old to start loving and celebrating life.

We are living in a wonderful time where old attitudes about aging are being thrown out and redefined. The idea that we are supposed to just sit somewhere and wait for our death after retirement has been turned on its head by defiant baby boomers who have decided that they will not stop working, learning or enjoying life. Instead, they are embracing the next phase of their lives with openness and anticipation. When I was growing up, we would often laugh with admiration at Celine, a distant relative who would occasionally come to visit my grandmother. In her old age, she was missing most of her teeth and it was hard to understand what she was saying most of the time. But she had this wonderful vigor and vitality. She walked everywhere and nothing seemed to stop her from going where she wanted to go.

In beauty may I walk...

In beauty, may I walk.

All day long, may I walk.

Through the returning seasons, may I walk.

On the trails marked with pollen, may I walk.

With grasshoppers about my feet, may I walk.

With dew about my feet, may I walk.

With beauty, may I walk.

With beauty before me, may I walk.

With beauty behind me, may I walk.

With beauty above me, may I walk.

With beauty below me, may I walk.

With beauty all around me, may I walk.

In old age wandering on a trail of beauty, lively, may I walk.

In old age wandering on a trail of beauty, living again, may I walk.

It is finished in beauty.

It is finished in beauty.

—NAVAJO PRAYER

Afterward

keep on walking

My hope is that you will keep walking with an open heart and mind, with a vibrant spirit, healthy body and radiant beauty.

As you write the next chapter on your path of wellness, know that you are worth the effort. Embracing the challenge to seek wellness opens the door to discover the deepest and highest intentions for our lives. We each have a unique path to walk, but we are in this together. We are making the world a better place when we commit to making ourselves happier and healthier beings who live with grace, gratitude and wisdom.

I hope that as you traverse and travel, you will continually renew and celebrate the beauty and greatness within and around you. If you have a setback or challenge, remember that this is a practice. We are not called to be perfect, but to be our highest selves, and that is a lifelong journey that doesn't always go as we plan. But returning to conscious commitment to staying connected to yourself and your source of energy will remind you that we are not alone on this journey. We are powerful, strong, creative and connected beings on a great adventure, seeking beauty, living beauty, being beauty!

suggested reading

Women's Bodies, Women's Wisdom: Creating Physical and Emotional Health and Healing by Christiane Northrup (Bantam Books, 2006).

Creating True Peace: Ending Violence in Yourself, Your Family, Your Community, and the World by Thich Nhat Hanh (Free Press, 2003).

A Return to Love: Reflections on the Principles of A Course in Miracles by Marianne Williamson (HarperCollins, 1992).

Your Life is Your Message: Finding Harmony With Yourself, Others, and the Earth by Eknath Easwaran (Hyperion, 1997)

Dealing with Depression Naturally: Complementary and Alternative Therapies for Restoring Emotional Health by Syd Baumel (Keats, 2000).

Jivamukti Yoga: Practices for Liberating Body and Soul by (Ballantine Books, 2002).

Perfect Health: The Complete Mind/Body Guide by Deepak Chopra (Harmony, 2001).

Finding Your Own North Star: Claiming the Life You Were Meant to Live by Martha Beck (Three Rivers Press, 2002).

How Much Does Your Soul Weigh?: Diet-Free Solutions to Your Food, Weight, and Body Worries by Dorie McCubbrey (Collins, 2004).

acknowledgments

First and foremost, I would like to thank God for the breath that I breathe, the inspiration to write this book, and the energy that sustained me through the entire process.

To Robert, I love and appreciate you. You are teaching me so much about love. Thank you for helping me "find my balance."

To Michelle Romelus, my creative editor, I am grateful for all that you do. Thank you for enthusiastically cheering me on and offering your honest opinion.

To my Dad, Mom, family and friends, thank you for your unwavering love and support.

To all the women who have attended or participated in Heart and Style programs and events, your commitment to your own health and wellbeing has affirmed and guided this work.

Many thanks to the women who contributed stories and ideas for this book. You remind us that health and balance is possible for every woman.

To my friend and colleague Terri Holley, you are an awesome health and life coach! I am grateful for your quick and thoughtful feedback.

Special thanks to Robin Quinn and Jo-Ann Langseth for your critique of my manuscript. Jo-ann, I appreciate your wit and encouragement.

To my editors, Ally Peltier and Henry Covey, I am so grateful I found you. Thank you for preserving my voice and words. It was a joy to work with both of you.

Kath Scheg, Elizabeth Crosgrove, Yuichi Miyoshi and the many others that help me stay "well"—you are healers, doing life-saving work. I bow to your greatness!

selected bibliography

Principle 1: Open Your Mind to Wellness

Zhi Gang Sha, *Soul Mind Body Medicine: A Complete Soul Healing System for Optimum Health and Vitality* (Novato: New World Library, 2006).

Barbara Loecher et al., "Imagery and visualization: using your mind's eye to heal" in *New Choices in Natural Healing for Women* (Emmaus: Rodale Press, 1997).

Howard LeWine, "Want to live longer? Think positive." *Newsweek.* http://www.msnbc.msn.com/id/6802862/site/newsweek/

Rob Stein, "Study is first to confirm that stress speeds aging," *Washington Post,* November 30, 2004, pg. A01.

A Course in Miracles (Mill Valley: Foundation for Inner Peace, 1992).

Rita and Blair Justice, "On giving: effects on the mind, body and soul," University of Texas Health Science Center *Health Leader.* http://www.healthleader.uthouston.edu/archive/Mind_Body_Soul/2003/ongiving-1222.html

Principle 2: Find Your Balance

Miranda Hitti, "Overtime work may be worse for women," *WebMD.* http://www.webmd.com/news/20060712/overtime-work-may-be-worse-for-women

CM Stoney, "Plasma homocysteine levels increase in women during psychological stress," *Life Sciences,* 64, 25 (1999): 2359-2365.

Jeannette Haviland-Jones, Holly Hale Rosario, Patricia Wilson, Terry McGuire, "An environmental approach to positive emotion: flowers," *Evolutionary Psychology,* 3 (2005): 104-132.

Society of American Florists, "Research shows flowers boost seniors' happiness, memory, social networks," Flowers and Seniors Study conducted by Jeannette Haviland-Jones, Rutgers University. http://www.aboutflowers.com/seniorstudy.htm

American Psychological Association, "Americans engage in unhealthy behaviors to manage stress." http://apahelpcenter.mediaroom.com/index.php?s=press_releases&item=23

Shelly Taylor et al., "Female responses to stress: tend and befriend, not fight or flight," *Psychological Review*, 107, 3 (2000): 411-429.

Klein L Cousino and EJ Corwin, "Seeing the unexpected: how sex differences in stress responses may provide a new perspective on the manifestation of psychiatric disorders," *Current Psychiatry Reports*, 4, No. 6 (2002): 441-448.

Thomas Rutledge et al., "Social networks are associated with lower mortality rates among women with suspected coronary disease: the National Heart, Lung, and Blood Institute-Sponsored Women's Ischemia Syndrome Evaluation Study," *Psychosomatic Medicine*, 66 (2004) 882-888.

Etienne Benson, "The many faces of perfectionism," *Monitor on Psychology*, 34, No. 10 (2003), pg. 18.

ScienceDaily, "Perfectionism can lead to imperfect health: high achievers more prone to emotional, physical and relationship problems." http://www.sciencedaily.com/releases/2004/06/040614074620.htm

L Bernardi, C Porta and P Sleight, "Cardiovascular, cerebrovascular, and respiratory changes induced by different types of music in musicians and non-musicians: the importance of silence," *Heart*, 92 (2006): 445-452.

Nancy Arcayna, "Music makes good medicine," *Honolulu Star Bulletin*. http://starbulletin.com/2006/07/18/features/story01.html

Principle 3: Nourish Your Spirit

Ronny Bell et al., "Prayer for health among U.S. adults: the 2002 national health interview survey," *Complementary Health Practice Review*, 10, No. 3 (2005) 175-188.

Stephen Kiesling, "The prayer war—Herbert Benson's research on health benefits of prayer," *Psychology Today*, October 1989.

Sharon Gannon and David Life, *Jivamukti Yoga: Practices for Liberating Mind,*

Body and Soul (New York: Ballantine Books, 2002).

National Institutes of Health, "More than one-third of U.S. adults use complementary and alternative medicine, according to new government survey," NIH News Advisory. http://nccam.nih.gov/news/2004/052704.htm

Luciano Bernardi et al, "Effect of rosary prayer and yoga mantras on autonomic cardiovascular rhythms: comparative study," British Medical Journal, 323 (2001) 22-29.

Joel Stein, "Just say om," Time Magazine. http://www.time.com/time/magazine/article/0,9171,1101030804-471136,00.html

Steve Caplan, "Standing out: Rodney Yee," Natural Awakenings, June 2006.

Jason Bartlett, "Americans filled with spirit, survey finds," The Penn Current, April 3, 2003.

Principle 4: Open Your Heart

Doc Childre and Howard Martin, The HeartMath Solution (New York: Harper-Collins, 1999).

Rollin McCraty, Raymond Trevor Bradley and Dana Tomasino, "The resonant heart," Shift, 5, (Dec. 2004-Feb. 2005): 15-19.

Michele Tugade, Barbara Fredrickson and Lisa Feldman Barret, "Psychological resilience and positive emotional granularity: examining the benefits of positive emotions on coping and health," Journal of Personality, 72, No. 6 (2004): 1161-1190.

Keiki Otake et el., "Happy people become happier through kindness: a counting kindnesses intervention," Journal of Happiness Studies, 7 (2006): 361-375.

Nancy Allison, "A brief history of journal therapy," in The Illustrated Encyclopedia of Mind-Body Medicine, (New York: The Rosen Publishing Group, 1999).

Joshua Smyth et al., "Effects of writing about stressful experiences on symptom reduction in patients with asthma or rheumatoid arthritis," JAMA, 281 (1999): 1304-1309.

Principle 5: Honor Your Body

Christiane Northrup, *Women's Bodies, Women's Wisdom: Creating Physical and Emotional Health and Healing* (New York: Bantam, 1998).

Barbara Howard and David Kritchevsky, "Phytochemicals and cardiovascular disease," *Circulation*, 95 (1997): 2591.

John Fauber, "Drink to your health?" *Milwaukee Journal Sentinel*. http://www.jsonline.com/story/index.aspx?id=440126

Brian Wansink and Kim Junyong, "Bad popcorn in big buckets: portion size can influence intake as much as taste," *Journal of Nutrition Education and Behavior*, 37, 5 (Sept-Oct 2005): 242-5.

Harvard School of Public Health Nutrition Source: http://www.hsph.harvard.edu/nutritionsource/

Katherine Combes, "Illness, the four seasons, and the four parts of the day," *The Epoch Times*, February 17, 2004.

Sari Van Anders, Elizabeth Hampson and Neil Watson, "Seasonality, waist-to-hip ratio, and testosterone," *Psychoneuroendocrinology*, 31 (2006) 895-9.

Deepak Chopra, *Perfect Health: The Complete Mind-Body Guide* (New York: Harmony Books, 1991).

National Heart, Lung and Blood Institute, "Your guide to healthy sleep," NIH publication, No. 06-5800, April 2006.

National Sleep Foundation, "Stressed out American women have no time for sleep," 2007 Sleep in America Poll, press release, March 6, 2007.

Shankar Vedantam, "Understanding that loving feeling," *The Washington Post*, July 29, 2002, A02.

index

about the author

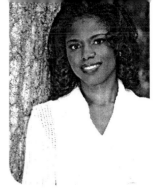

Judy Marjorie Lubin, MPH is a passionate writer, businesswoman, women's health and wellness advocate and the founder of Heart and Style, a lifestyle media company that inspires women to live healthy and fuller lives.

Judy is also president of Public Square Communications, a health communications and social marketing company that develops and manages innovative programs for reaching and empowering women, families and communities. She has served as an advisor and consultant to nationally recognized organizations and agencies, including the U.S. Department of Health and Human Services' Office on Women's Health and the Congressional Black Caucus Foundation. As a writer and health communications expert, Judy translates and distills health and medical information to inform and educate diverse audiences on how to take better care of their personal and family health. She has written for websites, television and radio on everything from women's health to childhood obesity to fashion and style. Judy and her work have been featured on national and local media including *Ebony Magazine*, *The Wall Street Journal*, *XM SatelliteRadio*, *NetPulse*, *Onyx Woman Magazine*, *Star Telegram* and *Observe* newspapers.

She has built an impressive track record for raising money, awareness, and support for some of today's most pressing women's, health and social issues. Judy has worked on national campaigns including the National Breastfeeding Awareness Campaign sponsored by the Ad Council and the Office on Women's Health and Super Sunday National Breast Cancer Awareness initiative. She is a former coordinator and facilitator for the National Minority AIDS Council's Women of Color Advocacy Program, an initiative designed to prepare participants to advocate for women affected by HIV/AIDS. A former coach for the Atlanta Avon Breast Cancer 3-Day, she successfully coached and supported over 400 women, helping to raise over $1 million dollars to support the Avon Foundation's breast cancer education, research and treatment programs. Judy has been honored by General Mills with a Cheerios Sisters Saving Hearts Award for her commitment to fighting heart disease among African American women.

A former Congressional Black Caucus Foundation Public Health Fellow and University of Tennessee, Knoxville Ronald McNair Scholar, Judy holds a Bachelor of Psychology from Florida State University (cum laude) and a Master of Public Health in Behavioral Sciences from Emory University. She is also a professionally trained wellness and intrinsic coach.

Judy regularly shares health and lifestyle news, ideas and resources on her website and blog, www.heartandstylewoman.com

heart and style™
www.heartandstylewoman.com

the
heart of
living well

Resource Guide

Visit heartandstylewoman.com to download the free companion resource guide, featuring tools and resources for each of the six principles. You'll also find information about Heart and Style's programs and events, opportunities to network with other health and socially-conscious women, plus the latest women's health news.

Log on today!

933692

Made in the USA